THE
YOGI CODE

THE
YOGI CODE

SEVEN UNIVERSAL LAWS
OF INFINITE SUCCESS

Yogi Cameron

ENLIVEN BOOKS
—
ATRIA

NEW YORK   LONDON   TORONTO   SYDNEY   NEW DELHI

ENLIVEN™

ATRIA

An Imprint of Simon & Schuster, Inc.
1230 Avenue of the Americas
New York, NY 10020

First Enliven Books/Atria Paperback edition May 2018

This publication contains the opinions and ideas of its author. It is intended to provide helpful and informative material on the subjects addressed in the publication. It is sold with the understanding that the author and publisher are not engaged in rendering medical, health, or any other kind of personal professional services in the book. The reader should consult his or her medical, health, or other competent professional before adopting any of the suggestions in this book or drawing inferences from it.

The author and publisher specifically disclaim all responsibility for any liability, loss, or risk, personal or otherwise, that is incurred as a consequence, directly or indirectly, of the use and application of any of the contents of this book.

For information about special discounts for bulk purchases, please contact Simon & Schuster Special Sales at 1-866-506-1949 or business@simonandschuster.com.

The Simon & Schuster Speakers Bureau can bring authors to your live event. For more information or to book an event, contact the Simon & Schuster Speakers Bureau at 1-866-248-3049 or visit our website at www.simonspeakers.com.

Interior design by Kyoko Watanabe

Manufactured in the United States of America

10 9 8 7 6 5 4 3 2 1

The Library of Congress has cataloged the hardcover edition as follows:
Names: Alborzian, Cameron, author.
Title: The yogi code : seven universal laws of infinite success / Yogi Cameron.
Description: New York : Enliven Books, [2017]
Identifiers: LCCN 2016039339 (print) | LCCN 2016044072 (ebook) | ISBN 9781501154522
    (hardcover) | ISBN 9781501154539 (pbk.) | ISBN 9781501154546 (eBook)
Subjects: LCSH: Yoga.
Classification: LCC BL1238.54 .A429 2017 (print) | LCC BL1238.54 (ebook) |
    DDC 204/.4—dc23
LC record available at https://lccn.loc.gov/2016039339

ISBN 978-1-5011-5452-2
ISBN 978-1-5011-5453-9 (pbk)
ISBN 978-1-5011-5454-6 (ebook)

To Yogini Jaima.

The divine shines through you wherever you go.

CONTENTS

CONTENTS

THE
YOGI CODE

Live Beyond the Ordinary

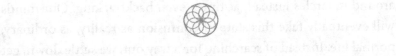

The journey of life is similar to a walk through a maze. We enter the world like everyone else, but instantly separate in different directions depending on the environment and family we are born into. At certain points, we come to junctions with two or three other paths; this is when we have to make a decision, deciding which direction to take without really knowing how long the journey will last or where it will lead.

Some push on through blindly by guessing. Many impulsively choose based on how they feel or their mood in the moment. Others come to an intellectual or practical decision based on logic and rationale. But very few choose to sit, close their eyes, contemplate, and listen to what their intuition or soul is directing them to do. And then, even fewer people have the inclination to follow this inner voice completely and wholeheartedly without allowing the mind to cast a shadow of a doubt.

By this stage most of us are now lost in this self-created maze of the mind due to all our past decisions and choices. This is where the mind becomes confused or stressed, because while it thought it was making progress forward, now it realizes it has been going around in circles instead, at times even backtracking. Our minds will eventually take this state of confusion as reality, as ordinary, normal life. Instead of searching for a way out, we settle down, get comfortable, and make a home in it.

We need our higher spiritual Self to guide our way out of this maze, to ignite our superconsciousness in order to have the capacity and wisdom to make the right decisions that lead to the exit—to liberation. This is what it means to take the "spiritual path," a path that is not heard or seen in the external, physical sense. Rather, it is invisible and within us. Science, medicine, and technology cannot find a way to the higher Self by inventing a device or a pill. They cannot build a powerful telescope or microscope to see it. The greatest of the scientific minds, such as Dr. Stephen Hawking, have made it their life's work to find answers to the question: "Why am I?" And they are still searching and will forever be searching until they turn inward. The theory of life and our universe cannot be answered by outward testing or material discoveries; it can be reached and answered through one way: *yogic spiritual practices.* And the one who can master these spiritual practices is the yogi.

These spiritual practices are the sounds, light, vibrations, movements, and images that form and come together in a specific and detailed manner to unlock and penetrate the higher consciousness. The yogi is the master who knows how to put these tools together in the correct configuration to make them open up and reveal the hidden secrets of our inner universe.

Who Can Become a Yogi?

The answer is anyone can become a yogi. The only difference is that a yogi not only lives by society's laws but lives and is guided by universal spiritual principles, written and taught by the ancient sages—the spiritual scientists and philosophers of their time. While modern scientists use outer matter to conduct experiments and to do studies to arrive at theoretical conclusions, yogis use their own body and mind as a lifelong experiment and prove their results through self-realization and personal experience. Life becomes a grand science project with a higher goal and purpose.

Through practices to control the body, breath, senses, and mind, yogis can start to remove the veil that separates their mind from their higher Self or soul. These practices are so subtle and powerful that they help transcend the body and mind into superconsciousness. The spiritual practices taught in this book are the principles and codes that will unlock and reveal the pathways to the next levels of transcendence and the invisible kingdom of the extraordinary. This level is where we act from our intuitive nature and not so much from our intellectual mind. In other words, we not only live by using our body and mind but we gain access to much greater powers to put toward our life's loves and pursuits, making them much more purposeful.

I wrote *The Yogi Code* so you could have the same essential tools that these ancient masters developed through centuries of practice and realization, passed down from generations of yogis to my yogi, and now from me to you. Once considered "secret knowledge," these seven universal laws are available to anyone who is ready to choose a new way of life—to illuminate your soul's purpose—promising harmony, success, and joy. These rewards are the outcomes, the fruits of your yogic life, that flow out of your conscientious practice and actions. As with anything in life, the more we practice, the better we get and the better the results.

The Yogi Code is an inspirational book to give you confidence and remind you that there is a greater universal plan than just the day-to-day life you are living. But inspiration is only the theoretical part of the practice—a beacon that shines a light, guiding and uplifting your mind and heart to show you the possibilities. However, the bulk of this content is much more than inspiration; it is a practical handbook that offers a new set of skills to learn, practice, and master.

All the inspiration in the world will not make you achieve something. When you break your arm, you don't get better simply by lying in bed and thinking positive thoughts. Progress and healing come through the practical guidance and rehabilitation the doctor or natural practitioner prescribes, so you can strengthen and learn to use your arm again. This is how these practices work in this book. In chapter 3, I've outlined the yogi code core practices—they are the foundational grounding practices for your body and your mind to be balanced while you interact with the world. In addition, at the end of every chapter, I've given you daily living practices to use as the need arises and to apply when the situation calls for them. When you make them a part of your daily life and lifestyle, you start to live as a yogi and move beyond your ordinary power.

Controlling faculties such as your breath, speech, actions, and senses brings your mind and body under your control, so you can move inward and create what is truly beautiful and meaningful. You build success from the inside out. This way you shine like the rare diamond that you are at the very core of your being, illuminating every step you take in life.

Once you start to live more as a yogi, your whole life will change beyond what you thought possible. Your personality, environment, work, relationships, and even some of your friends will change. This is all part of the process of transformation. But I know from my own experience that you will welcome and be energized by all the changes, because your life will have improved beyond all your expectations, and you will feel dynamically alive from within. The yogic path offers an exceptional journey that can lead to great power and fulfillment. It's like no other journey you will ever take.

When greeting others, place your hand
on your heart and say Namaste.

Activate Your Yogi Code

You don't need any special qualifications to become a yogi. You don't need to be part of an exclusive caste, club, or group. You don't need to drop your current life and relocate to a hermit's cave. All you need to do is start where you are.

The yogic life chooses you—you don't choose it. It requires an open mind-set and a yearning from deep within your soul, something within driving and pulling you in a certain direction that you have no real control over. Everything that happens in your life is a prelude, drawing you closer and deeper onto the path even if you are currently in a whole other seemingly unconnected world or lifestyle.

Lahiri Mahasaya, the great kriya yogi, had an office job as an accountant and later was posted at a mountain military site, as recounted in the epic stories told by Indian guru and yogi Paramahansa Yogananda in his beautiful book *Autobiography of a Yogi*. It was there that he met his guru, Babaji, and went on the yogic path, creating a lineage and legacy of generations of yogis in India to this day. Every bit of his life had been preparing and leading him to take that journey. He was a regular person living a "regular" life just like you.

In my own trajectory growing up in Iran, who knew I would end up on the yogic path as a yogi? I was living a "regular" family life with my mother and father when the revolution and war began in 1979. My mother rushed me out of the country to avoid being deployed to the front lines at the age of twelve. I landed in England, and within a few weeks was placed in a boarding school, even though I could not read or write English. My mother immediately returned to Iran to be with my father. I was on my own, dislocated from home and family, until my parents could find a way to safely leave Iran. I wouldn't see my father for four years and only saw my mother periodically when she could come and visit a couple of times a year.

I continued from boarding school to college for a year and then dropped out and headed to London to try my luck at any job I could get. I was nineteen, and my family was not pleased with my decision; they worried I would stay adrift. However, within a few weeks, while I was walking down one of London's hippest streets, a modeling agent scouted me. I soon ended up on the catwalks of Paris, Milan, and New York.

I traveled the world for twelve years, working and becoming friends with some of the most famous people on the planet and landing exclusive jobs, like appearing in Madonna's "Express Yourself" music video and being on the covers of fashion magazines like *Vogue* and *GQ*.

Never in my life would I have guessed I would become a model and be named one of the most famous supermodels of my time. It would seem my life had reached a pinnacle and couldn't get any better. The life of a supermodel is probably regarded as the most exciting, carefree, and glamorous life anyone can live; you make lots of money and people revere you as a beauty symbol. Life couldn't get much better on the outside. But what about the inside?

What I didn't know then was that I was at a crossroads, and the next chapter of my life was about to begin. Everything before had been preparation for something beyond my imagination—destiny would lead me to the extraordinary.

*

I had traveled from New York to Cape Town, South Africa, for a fashion show for Versace at Nelson Mandela's home. Upon my arrival at the hotel, I saw my friends and fellow models Kate Moss, Christy Turlington, and Naomi Campbell, and a few other well-known faces. It was like any other day on the job, nothing out of the ordinary.

We were scheduled to meet the president at the Palace Gardens the next day as well as prepare for the fashion show. That morning the atmosphere was both calm and electric as we stood in the receiving line and moved one at a time, as security didn't allow people to gather around Mandela. When it was my turn, I approached him to shake his hand. To know a person you look at their face; to know their soul you look into their eyes. I gazed deeply into Nelson Mandela's eyes. I don't remember what we spoke of; I just remember his eyes, sensing a silent exchange.

The gathering was over a few hours later, and we proceeded to a dress rehearsal and fitting. The house of Versace makes high fashion in a very colorful and extravagant way, so I knew it was going to be a spectacular event. I was excited and looking forward to the fun. Later that evening, there would be a private party.

When I woke up the next morning, something felt different. I couldn't place it, but I felt something within coming to the edge of my awareness. Before I could explore any further, I was distracted by the day's events. The show was amazing, and the glamorous after-party was filled with VIP guests from all over the world. It continued until the morning, and after a couple of hours of sleep, I was on the plane and headed home. Three days had gone by like a flash.

Back in New York, I reflected on my time in Cape Town. I recalled all the amazing moments, extreme excitement, beauty, glamour, and fame. And then I remembered meeting Nelson Mandela. Here was a soul who had it tough all his life; he courageously fought for freedom and basic human rights. He went to prison for twenty-seven years and came out smiling. In his eyes that night, I saw that his soul had always been free, although he had spent years in prison. I didn't see those walls being a hindrance; on the contrary, the prison was part of his soul's evolution. The prison had given strength to his soul to master a freedom that could not be taken away or lost; it did not control the spiritual freedom he had within. I came to see and understand that this experience of imprisonment and liberation was part of all of our paths—the need to be spiritually free and find our purpose.

I had arrived at a crossroads sparked by meeting Mandela and reflecting on his life. From my viewpoint as an observer, I wondered where I fit in. I started to see how on one side, I was living my outer beauty. It was an exciting life and fulfilling on many levels, especially for sensory pleasures. It was a life that very quickly met most of my desires. I thought: *Maybe this is why I'm seeing my life differently now. Have I had all my desires met? What more is there to achieve in fashion?* On the other side, I felt something more powerful pulling me toward it, but I didn't know what that journey was yet. All I felt was its undeniable force, which I wasn't quite ready to surrender to.

So what was my purpose? This was the question I was exploring at this new crossroads in my life, and I had to decide which path to take. I decided to alight from the fashion ride at the next stop, but without knowing my true destination. What I was sure about was I needed to get off. I couldn't control the "wherever," but I could control the "whenever," so I took that action right away.

I retired from modeling, and after a few years of wandering and searching, I ended up in India training in the sciences of yoga and ayurveda. Ayurveda is the traditional Indian medicine that comes from the oldest books of knowledge: the Vedas. And now, some fourteen years later, I live part of my life as a yogi in a rain forest in India and spend the other part traveling and sharing yogic teachings with people around the world.

If anyone had looked into the future and explained to me that this was going to be my life, I might have had a hard time imagining it. Mine is definitely not a common spiritual path! But then again, spirituality doesn't discriminate against professions or people; it is available to anyone who chooses to follow it. And at times, even if you don't choose it, the spiritual path often prods until you surrender and do.

When I first left Iran, my only wish was to stay with my family. I remember being dropped off by my mother at boarding school in the north of England. As she drove away, just one tear slid down my cheek, and that was the end of my pain. I had a wonderful time at school, and I barely missed my family from then on. Something within me was totally okay with being alone. I had an intuitive feeling that I was taken care of and that things would always be fine.

Looking back, I can see how this experience of early separation from my family was preparing me for the yogic life. My past *karma* (actions) was steering me through what I had to experience as part of my spirit's journey and purpose.

I also learned that it's best not to expect someone to be solely there for you, even if they want to, because ultimately at times circumstances dictate our situations. Maybe at best we can depend on others to assist, but relying on someone to always be there for your needs is a risk that can steer you outside of your life's purpose (as well as the other person, who has his or her own life's purpose).

I learned early on to trust the voice from within, although I wasn't fully conscious of where this voice was coming from at the time; it would become my guiding star to the yogi path.

When the Yogi Is Ready, the Path Will Appear

A yogi is quite detached in his being, and this was my training from an early age. I spent a lot of my young adult life alone, focused on my modeling career, until I met Ron, who would become my best friend and spiritual mentor, in Paris.

One day in the gym, I saw a man who appeared to be in his forties or fifties wearing a green tracksuit and headband and looking at me with a cheerful, friendly smile. I introduced myself to him, and we started talking like we'd known each other a hundred years. After some weeks of regular chatting, we learned a lot about each other. I found out that Ron had contracted HIV.

With my growing friendship with him, a new part of my life

began. By day, I was shooting magazine covers for *GQ* in Milan, doing advertising for Guess jeans and Versace on location in Hawaii, and filming music videos for Elton John in London. But on my days off and at night I was mainly hanging out with Ron.

He introduced me to the study of spirituality, guiding me through his own knowledge and experiences. He had me read a diverse range of books on spirituality from the 1960s and 1970s and took me to seminars by Deepak Chopra and Marianne Williamson, when she was teaching *A Course in Miracles*. At nineteen I was leading a dual lifestyle—model by day, spiritual seeker by night. Then in 1998, I decided to leave the fashion business after meeting Nelson Mandela.

When I first met Ron, I would not have viewed him as a mentor. I realized he was more like a mentor to me only after he passed away fourteen years later. While he was alive, he was just my best friend. I remember us walking around Paris all the time hand in hand or arm in arm, chatting away about life. Most people thought we were in a romantic relationship, because they saw me everywhere with this older man. We found this very amusing, and even played it up at times just to keep people guessing. It was fun, especially because I had a girlfriend, which made people even more curious and confused. My mother is English, and most of my childhood was spent in that culture where our "English sense of humor" is just this way.

I learned from early on that when a young man has an older

gay male friend or teacher, the world will comment, have opinions, and judge, but that was okay with me. It was all part of the process of being both an individual and part of the whole. Ron taught me never to react and to allow others to have their opinions, but always try and live by what was true in me. It was an extremely valuable lesson that has been with me ever since. It allowed me to be comfortable with myself and leave others to be themselves— no judgment, no reaction. Ours was a true and loving friendship between two beings who enjoyed spending time together—it was my experience of a deep and caring friendship.

Spirituality and the quest to reach our purpose were our common goals and favorite topics of discussion to the very end of his life. I remember looking into his eyes shortly before he left his body and seeing the same thing I saw in Mandela's eyes. He was free and had completed his purpose.

After Ron's death, I left Paris and went to New York. I wanted to expand on what we had been discussing all those years, but again, I wasn't sure how to go about it. Although I had been practicing yoga and living a pretty healthy life, I didn't think I had been using what I'd learned in a daily practice. I was a casual spiritualist.

In early 2003, I trained for six months in yoga teacher training at Integral Yoga Institute in New York. This was a good start to walking the yogic path, but I felt I needed much more knowledge on the subject. I had read a book by Dr. David Frawley called *Yoga & Ayurveda*, which explains how the two sciences are practiced together according to the teaching of the ancient *rishis,* or sages, of India. This was my missing link.

Frawley says that ayurveda is the science of the body, while yoga is the science of the mind and beyond. This is exactly what I was beginning to experience, and I realized that I needed to go to the source of these two sciences to evolve more deeply on this path. In more than fifteen years of trotting around the globe, I never had the urge to visit India, the land of spirituality. Now I know why: I was not ready to meet my teachers until I had done some prior work to prepare myself for what was to come.

Two weeks after I finished my teacher training in New York City, I traveled to India, where I met and went to school under the guidance of my guru, Sri Vasudevan. When I say *guru,* I should explain that at times it means teacher and at other times it means guide. This can apply to a variety of people in your life, but a guru who is enlightened and can leave the physical body at will is something else entirely. This higher being has given up control in order for his soul to be completely in charge of his body and life, and these are rare beings you will not meet under normal circumstances. My guru is a teacher and guide. I have yet to encounter my enlightened guru and master. This will come at my next stage of spiritual training.

I understood these spiritual teachings were not easy to grasp and were even more difficult to put into practice unless I had a guru to lead the way. I also came to understand that the "outer guru" is a reflection of our own "inner guru" that is also teaching and guiding us. The outer guru guides us to the point where we can learn to follow the inner guru.

With guidance and years of study and practice, I realized that not only did I want to teach this path, I wanted to devote my life to it and live as a true yogi. This is when I went from "Cameron" to "Yogi Cameron." After making my commitment, along with receiving more training and guidance from my teachers, I was finally ready and was allowed to teach. I was instructed that it was time to go back to America to share this knowledge with those who wanted to become yogis or to apply these practices to their daily lives.

At first I was a little uncomfortable with this instruction. I liked the life of meditation in India, so I suggested I stay longer—or even forever! "And if you stay, what are you going to do here?" asked my guru. I hadn't thought this through, so I said unconvincingly, "Practice and learn more!"

We both knew it was time for me to leave and start to share the practices and knowledge, but my resistance in going back to Western society stemmed from the fact that it was a very extreme and abrupt change of environment and lifestyle. I had already lived the high and fast life as a model, and now I was at the other end of the spectrum, living slow and simple. Going from a small Indian village to the big city seemed to be moving between two extremely different and opposing worlds.

How was I going to do this? I was once a well-known model, but that was more than ten years ago, and I no longer had any kind of public presence. Most people outside of India didn't even know what a yogi was or how he lived. How was a fashion model turned yogi going to be taken seriously? How would people understand? The whole idea sounded a little outlandish, even to an open-minded person.

I realized it didn't matter what other people thought, or what my mind was resisting. I only had to trust in my spiritual practice, my commitment to the wisdom and training I had learned from my guru, and follow my intuition—the yogi within me would guide me on the path ahead. This is when my training moved from theory into practice.

The Spiritual Roots of the Yogi Code

The science of true yoga teaches that the longing we feel deep inside is the spirit of cosmic consciousness—the divine spirit, God, universe, or any other name you wish to give it. Yoga teaches us that the separation we think is there only exists in our mind, because our eyes are fixed on the material outer world, which has us mesmerized and distracted. Just like a movie, it seems real because of the visual images, but our intellect knows it is all just an illusion and plays along, suspending disbelief.

Therefore, the idea behind spiritual yogic practices is to turn our focus inward, removing the illusion that we only need the outer material world, and instead move into a universe much more immense and endless than the outer world we exist in momentarily. This means true liberation beyond the body, where there is no physical or mental suffering.

This liberation from the veil of the material world and its suffering is the inspiration and purpose behind the teachings of *The Yogi Code*, which have been selected from the Vedic knowledge system. The original ancient texts where yoga and ayurveda come from are called the Vedas, comprised of four vast volumes of work, which are not easy for the layperson to comprehend but are written for the devout spiritual seeker. Within these sacred volumes are all the secrets of yoga and ayurveda, as well as the spiritual laws we need to live by to understand and conquer death. All yogic paths lead from the Vedas and back to them. They are the beginning and the end of all spiritual knowledge.

I selected these seven yogic laws or principles especially for the times we live in. We are in the age of technology and speed. People are moving faster, and time seems to be moving more quickly. Everyone seems to need more time, but can't find it in their lives to reach their goals. More people are struggling with stress or depression or feeling overwhelmed, and are taking a lot of medication to cope. People are lost as to what their purpose is, living in constant overdrive. These modern-day issues, evident for so long in the industrialized world, have been growing more common throughout the nonindustrialized world as well.

On a trip to Cambodia, I was speaking to an office manager from a charitable foundation who told me, "We know soda and junk food are really bad for us, but we want to be modern, live modern, think modern, and become a developed country quickly so we are not considered a third-world country anymore." I saw the same thing happening when I was teaching in China and India. Excess has become the new "normal," and along with it have come most of our health problems and spiritual confusion.

The ancient seers saw and knew the turbulent age we would be living in, so to help us through these difficult and challenging times, they devised practices to help us live with integrity, kindness, and compassion—our higher consciousness. As you learn these yogic practices and make them part of your daily life, you will become a seer and a yogi too. Your point of view, your attitude, and your actions will all become clear, peaceful, and loving. Compassion becomes your nature and joy becomes a way of life. You start to embody truth and leave fear behind. The yogi is a practitioner and eventually a leader on the spiritual path.

When we are fixated on the outer world and invest all our time thinking about things such as money, career, relationships, success, and belongings, our minds become engrossed in our surroundings through the senses. In this mental state, we only believe in a material existence, and all other levels of consciousness stay out of reach or unknown to us.

Our society is focused on machines and technology, thinking

the more we see progress on these material levels the more we are advancing as humans. But we need to look back at our progress so far. Have we been able to live peacefully, lovingly, or kindly with others and the environment for the last five thousand years? We are advancing by leaps and bounds on the technological front, but on all other levels of humanity and spirituality, we are sinking deeper and deeper into an abyss of ignorance, cruelty, and fear, trying to protect ourselves from the "enemy"—namely other people. The only real enemy is the fear we have created inside our minds.

It's time to shift our focus from the material world and end our self-inflicted suffering and stress. It's time to return to that from which we came, the cosmic consciousness of our universe that connects all beings together. We can either come together, being our most loving and compassionate selves, or we can continue to live disconnected and in fear of one another, pointing out our differences such as race, religion, sexual orientation, and political views. One path leads to liberation and purpose on the highest level, and the other keeps us stuck exactly where we are, on a much lower one. It's time to choose your path—no one can exist on both.

How to Activate Your Inner Yogi

We read a lot about successful people and their life stories, their struggles and their ups and downs. But usually there is a common thread in how they made it: a lot of determination and persistency in their dreams and beliefs. We live in a world where we define successful people as the ones who build empires and companies that are worth billions. They are people who hold world records and win championships, who have fame and wealth, who have gone beyond the ordinary and become the few celebrated ones.

We also recognize others who have overcome disease, disability, hardship, or extreme struggle through poverty or addiction. These are examples not necessarily of successful people, but of inspirational people, people we look up to who never gave up and overcame the odds.

But it isn't often that we think about being healthy in body, mind, and spirit as being successful. We don't associate having a balanced and calm mind as successful, or being healthy as an accomplishment. There are no special contests or awards for this. But not getting sick and keeping a healthy body and mind is the backbone of any spiritually successful person. Can a person go to work, tend to their children with a healthy attitude, be of use to anyone if they are sick in bed?

Our health on all levels of body and mind needs to be protected and preserved through a healthy lifestyle in order for us to achieve everything else we want to achieve in this lifetime. From the yogic prospective, a person who has health in body, mind, and spirit is the true definition of success.

To help you achieve this level of health and well-being, this book offers seven universal laws that, when followed and applied to your life, will guide you to become the most successful person you can be. Why is this? Because the success I'm defining is not limited to material, exterior success, which everyone puts so much emphasis on. This is often the most basic level of success: make a lot of money, have your desires met, and make your mark on this world. We have endless examples of people doing this. But what we don't have much of is balanced beings living in a healthy body and a peaceful mind, with spiritual purpose. This is the promise and outcome of dedicating yourself to these practices.

And once you have achieved this level of abundant success, how do you maintain it? So much emphasis is put on becoming successful and reaching our highest potential, but little is taught about being able to sustain this level of success. This is what you will learn as you work with these seven universal laws. So when life is not going your way, when challenges strike, instead of feeling lost and confused, you have the resilience and fortitude to feel complete and to keep moving forward without being distracted by your fears.

Your success will come from an inner source of power that nothing can shake or steal, and you won't be dependent on material objects or people to sustain your contentment. This is true freedom for the yogi.

The universal laws taught in this book invite you to redefine your story of success and take charge of who you are. By taking charge of your decisions and actions, your mind and senses, you activate the yogi within. These seven laws are:

1. **Routine:** This defines the way you live each day.
2. **Practice:** This gives you the tools to develop a unshakable spiritual foundation.
3. **Self-study:** This gives you the knowledge of who you really are and not who you have become.
4. **Intention:** This unearths your deepest desires that lie in your soul, which may be different from your spoken intentions.
5. **Purpose:** The biggest question anyone can contemplate; even if you gain everything you ever wanted, if your purpose is not lived, you feel an inner void.
6. **Service:** Cultivating an attitude of serving others and the world in all that we do and say brings a level of spirituality to our lives that is not reached through any other means.
7. **Love:** The culmination of all the other six practices will lead to a true, everlasting, and uninterrupted flow of love's energy; to experience this love, the mind will need to surrender itself to a greater awareness within.

Each of the following chapters is dedicated to one principle, offering both inspiration and practice for you to experience and integrate into your daily life. The secret to staying on the yogic path is sustained practice of these spiritual principles. The ancient sages have said that the mind and body can only be fully controlled through three steps:

1. Practice done for a long time
2. Practice without breaks
3. Practice with full attention and in all earnestness

This is how the essence and purpose of the yogi is unveiled over time. To discover the bigger truths and higher meaning of your life, you have to uncover the secrets to spirituality and live them through daily practice. The spiritual path is at times called a secret because it is hidden from the one who doesn't have the code to unearth it yet. To get to our higher inner power we need to practice continuously without distractions and for a long time. In other words, we need to practice daily and make it a part of our lifestyle.

✳

Often people ask me if I think they are spiritual, while others tell me how spiritual they are. Everyone relates to spirituality, but people don't always know how to connect to it. After all, telling people there is a universe within them is a nice thought and sounds like a beautiful idea, but to actually make it a reality as a self-realized experience takes practice. This is the level of the process that fewer people ever reach, but those who do are living with a different quality of life beyond the material or mental levels. This is where the universe of spirituality opens, and the "outer universe" appears so insignificant in comparison. You can be any kind of person—a felon or a saint. You can be a model or movie star. You can be a CEO or a politician. These are only job descriptions and not what is under the skin of the individual—the soul.

Spirituality is connecting with the soul and knowing your purpose—this is where life goes from ordinary to exceptional.

Routine: The Key to Healthy Habits

I lost my way for a few years after leaving the fashion world, thinking the gods might look down, take pity on me, and hand me another very successful career as a present. That never happened. In fact, because they gave me such a free ride to do as I pleased for more than a decade, it was now payback time—time to work hard and get very little in return for a while. Karma!

With no effort, I was handed my first career, and now I would have to work hard for the next eleven years to build a new one from scratch. The fact I didn't know what that particular career was yet made me feel somewhat confused. It is one thing to try and build a business when you know what that business is, but when you have no idea what direction your life will take, you feel like a lost cause.

By this time, I had spent most of my savings from my modeling days, which was fast becoming a threat to my survival. I was also a single father raising my young daughter, so her welfare was paramount, increasing my worries while I was trying to find my new path in the world. It's a funny thing how quickly you can go from being on top of the world as a celebrity and beauty symbol to having little money and not being treated as a hot commodity. It seemed to happen in just the blink of an eye.

On my first day of training at Integral Yoga Institute in New York, I found my new path. I felt for the first time since my retirement from modeling that I had found my missing spark, which would eventually ignite a fire and lead me somewhere. Looking back now, I see how my intuition had led me to pursue this yoga training; there was a natural ease to the work and the message resonated in me. The work brought me introspection and into deep contemplation even through the training was difficult, especially the postures, which were hard for my stiff body to perform. But this physical challenge was just part of the process of forming new habits, and besides, it was only one challenge out of my other bigger challenges to overcome.

One of these was how to be both a single parent and a yoga practitioner, taking care of my daughter's needs from early in the morning and through the day on one hand, and adhering to my new yoga routine on the other. I was supposed to get up early, maybe around six or seven, and begin my practice. First of all, I had to get over my not liking to wake up early, which usually resulted in a "forced" wake-up from my daughter at seven. That was my normal routine, and now with all my yogic practices, I had to look at my morning habits and intentionally make time for my practices. How was I going to attend to my daughter and follow the yogic path?

Getting up at 5:00 A.M. wasn't an option, as I would be sleep-walking if I attempted to rise at that time! I decided to wake up at 6:30 A.M., just thirty minutes before my daughter would get up, to get some practice in, adding one or two other practices to my daily routine. It would take quite a few years of being patient with my physical body, slowly becoming more flexible, and then a couple of years before I could adapt and continue to adjust to the many new habits required by the yogic path.

I had definitely found my path in life, but none of it was easy. It all came with a struggle. I remember pushing my daughter in her stroller in the noisy and busy streets of New York in the dead of winter with all the rain and snow, or in the extreme heat of the summer, and wondering when life was going to ease up a little and give me a break. It still hasn't. I learned to change my point of view and expectations that life is supposed to be easy or that it owes me something, and I learned to take responsibility for making the changes to my habits and routines that I needed to do to be both the kind of parent I wanted for my daughter and the yogi I was training to become.

*

What does it mean to have a routine? Basically anything you do daily and in a consistent manner is part of your routine. The activities that make up your daily routine are partly for your survival (sleeping, eating) and partly out of necessity (work or school), and then others are added from your desires or interests (exercise, entertainment, sports). The routines we have for our survival are quite fixed, but they can be continuously worked on to form better habits for us to live a more healthy and balanced life. The routines that come from necessity can always be perfected through greater awareness and being conscious of our limits and boundaries. The routines that come from our desires and interests are changeable, but are often the most challenging for us to adjust because we have a strong attachment to them.

It is our attachments that make change difficult.

Years ago, when people had very simple routines and lived off the land in tribes, life was a lot more straightforward. They understood their individual duties as well as their obligations to their community, which were all mainly for a common goal—survival. People didn't have any need for entertainment or the inclination for a lot of comfort, so their desire level was also much lower and closer to nature rather than being overstimulated by artificial machines and electronics. Today, in the name of freedom, we have decided that we should be able to choose anything we want, at any time, and with whomever we feel like. This has contributed to our desires getting out of our control to the point where we have a constant need for more, especially when it comes to new pleasures. Many of these habits we hold on to as part of our routine tend to be harmful to our life and are major contributors to the deterioration of our physical and mental health. Our desires also create habits that lead to pollution of both our inner and outer environments, a source of our breakdowns in communities and our feelings of oneness.

The ancient yogic texts such as the Vedas were written by self-realized sages to assist people in following a *satvic,* or more balanced, way of living in accordance with nature. These sages observed nature and the seasons, learning from the ultimate teacher, our earth. The balance of air, water, sun, and food was created perfectly to serve our bodies and minds. Our bodies were designed to support and sustain life in the particular part of the world where we lived, in that particular environment, and with that particular climate. But from the Industrial Revolution to our twenty-first-century lifestyles and technology, our nature and nature itself have both been forced out of balance.

To follow a yogic life is to once again find balance in our routines, so that we live in accordance with and relation to nature. The inherent wisdom of our ancient sages saw that without living in harmony with the natural world, the human world risks losing its true humanity.

Looking at Your Routine

As yogis, we start to look at our daily routine and observe it to see what is serving our purpose and what isn't. As we are trying to create balance in all aspects of our life, any habits that move us away from our healthy goals and spiritual aspirations will need to be altered. If you keep irregular habits and routines, your mind will not become consistent and peaceful. For instance, if one day you go to bed at 9:00 P.M., then another day you retire at 1:00 A.M., or if you eat dinner at 6:00 P.M. and then another night at 9:00 P.M., you are not creating a consistent pattern for your mind to commit to. The mind and body are like children—they need a routine, and when they don't have one they behave in an irritated way.

You also need to consider this question: What is more important to you at this stage of your development? Is staying up and having the "freedom" of an irregular sleeping schedule more important to you than starting to change your old pattern and going to sleep between 9:30 and 10:00 P.M. every night? Whatever is most important to you will always win your attention over everything else. For this reason you have to first contemplate why you even want to change this habit if you are going to stand a chance of shifting out of it for good.

Too many extreme inconsistencies and irregularities in our routine make for many different imbalances in our mind and body. But it's a personal choice to follow one routine or another. I work with many people who ask me how they can change their habit of sleeping late or lack of energy or being distracted. The answer is simple—choice.

Every time you choose to do something, it is the start of a habit. If you like to drink a glass of wine once a week, it is still a habit, even if it's a lesser one than that of the person who drinks once a day. Habits are habits. It is the frequency of them that causes us to lose control, but choice is involved—the choice to stop or continue the habit. It all ultimately depends on what your intention is for wanting to drink. When you want to alter, modify, or even change a habit completely, the alternative choice has to become more important than the desire to continue with the old habit.

When I first decided to embark on the yogic path, many of my habits needed changing and others needed to end completely. These included habits like staying up late, getting up when I liked, eating at any time, socializing in situations where frivolous or unproductive conversations were taking place, watching violent movies, and eating artificial sugars and foods. I had to cut all of these things out. With these choices went certain options and people, as they did not fit into my choices for a new lifestyle as a yogi. These were all part of a choice to change, because following the path was more important to me than my old lifestyle and the people and things that came with it.

Committing fully to the yogic path is not for everyone. It demands time, commitment, and discipline beyond the ordinary level. This is why it is more balanced of you to change and alter the things you are willing to at the present moment, and not to do more than you are willing. Overdoing things will only discourage you and make you more likely to give up, especially after the initial enthusiasm of starting on this path has faded.

When I first started doing yoga postures, I remember how stiff I was. It felt like it was going to take a hundred years for me to be able to touch my toes. And it really did take about ten years to slowly open my body up; even now and probably for the rest of my life, keeping my body from becoming stiff again will be a constant daily challenge. When I started each step on this path, I took up as much as I could handle at that time and slowly built on it; I continue to build on my practices to this very day and will keep on doing so. I am doing more than I did fifteen years ago, but not as much as I will be in the next fifteen. I am at present doing about three hours of daily practice, and this amount fits naturally and is in balance with my lifestyle.

Only you can choose what amount of change and time you put into your practice—take the steps that feel in harmony with where you are right now, which may mean a minimal step to begin with or perhaps a bigger one. See your life as a long-term journey and not just quick moments that keep passing by. Viewing your life not as hours and weeks but as years and lifetimes removes any anxiety to rush through life trying to do as much as possible as quickly as possible.

Routine of Spirituality

For the one who wants to go on the yogic path, life can be slightly different or vastly different. It just depends on how much of the path and practices you take on and make a part of your lifestyle. For people not on the yogic path, their routine is comprised mostly of things they have chosen for themselves. They live and reap the rewards or disappointments of their choices. They identify with certain religious, political, and personal beliefs that their family, friends, or partner may also follow. Their routine is mostly self-serving or self-motivated: to be able to enjoy life, make lots of money, have the perfect job, have status, and find pleasure with things in the world like having a family or finding the love of their life. Being as comfortable as possible in life is usually one of their major goals. The meaning of their existence and the purpose of life are usually a passing thought or a topic of discussion but not daily contemplation. And death is something morbid or negative that doesn't need discussing or thinking about too often.

For the yogi, everything above is exactly reversed, and the order of importance is changed. The pursuit of enlightenment and liberation from the body is of primary importance, with all other things coming after that. This pursuit is at the forefront of our minds because leaving the body and moving on from this life is a reality we need to be prepared for. It is a moment of great importance when we want to put our focus on a higher truth and not fear.

If a yogi can attain self-realization in this lifetime, they will know the time and day when it is the right moment to leave the body so the spirit can move beyond the earthly plain. The reason this is so important beyond all other things in a yogi's life is because it is taught by the ancient texts that when we leave the body we want to utter the name of the divine with our last breath. This is to help the soul drop any earthly attachments and move on without carrying any burdens from this life, which is what ultimate liberation feels like.

The routine one has to follow needs to reflect what the yogic texts teach so we can reach this goal. If you want to follow some of the teachings to benefit your life and change some of your habits, a routine overhaul is necessary to a certain degree. It's no good trying to follow more than you are willing to do or less than you are capable of. But the right amount is established by your determination and not always by your capabilities, which may be a lot more than your willpower.

A Day in the Life of a Yogi

Here is a glimpse of how I now start the day as a yogi:

The first step is to get up before sunrise. In winter months this should be at least by 5:30 A.M. even if the sun rises later. The timing can vary a little depending on my work schedule and how much rest I need. After brushing my teeth and taking a shower, I cleanse the body through purification practices called *shatkarmas*. Some of these practices include drinking and regurgitating of saltwater, cleansing the nasal passages, and rolling the stomach from side to side. Oiling the body, head, and all the orifices of the body is next. Then I practice several yoga postures to open the body for flexibility, which helps prepare me to sit on the floor in a cross-legged position. The sitting meditation is the most important aspect of the yogic path, and the other yoga movements are only a prelude—no one ever became spiritual or enlightened by only doing yoga postures.

Breathing practices are next, which help us to control the most powerful force in our body, *prana*, which is Sanskrit for vital life force. At the beginning stages this will help slow down our heart rate, normalize our blood pressure, and bring stillness to our system. At a more advanced stage these pranayama practices will break though different barriers of our psyche and give us control of our breathing by making it voluntary.

Then I perform some exercises to subdue and control my senses from outer influences: what I hear, see, touch, taste, and smell. Our senses are so stimulated and sensitive to outer distractions that controlling them through a disciplined lifestyle is essential if we want to experience the benefits of these yogic practices.

Once my body is settled in, my breath is under control, and my senses have been subdued, I am ready for concentration or meditation practices. From this stillness and introspection, I start to hear my inner guide, and my intuition starts to pull me inward. I lose the mental chatter and swim into conscious bliss. This is spontaneous meditation.

After meditation, I read some spiritual material to help me

through my day and keep me grounded in higher living. The energy and grounding that I have created through all of these morning practices are now taken into the rest of my day.

This is where the essence of my practice is used for my interactions and communication with the outer world. My whole approach to everything in life comes from this morning practice: my attitude, manner of speaking, and intentions. The practice for the day is to then breathe spiritual energy into every decision and action I take. I may be writing, having a meeting, doing an interview, filming, consulting, traveling, or doing any other activities that make up my day or week; whatever it is, I make it an extension of the energy created through the morning practice. I choose the work I do, the projects I get involved with, and the people I interact with based on what intentions I have set through my practice.

To close out my day, I usually see what is needed in the moment. Sometimes I sit an hour before bed and contemplate my day and my actions. This gives me insight into and awareness of what kind of energy I am creating, so I can adjust my actions according to what I want to attract. Other times I sit for some silent introspection, or I do some internal chanting, keeping this practice going into my sleep and dreams. What I don't do is read or stimulate the mind in any way, which will disturb my peace as I am getting ready for sleep.

*

These practices are the routine for a yogi, and it's a routine that is built step by step, practicing and integrating each component into a seamless movement that becomes a way of life. By practicing these daily yogic activities, you strengthen your inner guidance and intuition in order to be fearless in your outer life and have perfect clarity in your actions. You will know instinctively what to do next, and you will have answers to questions that need answering. You refresh and recharge your spiritual energy, and you move forward with intention and purpose. It's as if a window that was fogged up has cleared, and you can now see the road ahead.

Prepare to Live Beyond Your Limits

As you will see in the next chapter on practice, you will learn where your starting point is as a beginner, or if you are a seasoned practitioner, how you can enhance and expand your practice. No one jumps in and starts where I am. I didn't start where my teachers were when I began, or even when I had been practicing for many years. The key to practice is to create balance, not stress.

You will learn the art of timing, knowing when the time comes to add more, but never too soon. From my experience with my clients there are usually three different types of practitioners: the first one is inconsistent in their practice, so they don't ever feel they are receiving the full benefits of their practice; and the second one has tried too many different practices and becomes confused about what works best for them. It is rare to meet the third kind of practitioner, the one who practices daily and consistently for many years on the same path—with steadfastness, commitment, and persistency.

If you choose to commit to the yogic path, remember that you set the pace, striking the right balance of how much change you can take on and how much practice you integrate into your daily routine. It's not about diving in fast, looking for immediate results; it's not about doing it all at once.

As you add more practices and live fully on this path, you have less interest in distractive conversations, people, and actions. You have a natural tendency to move toward simpler and more meaningful conversations, people, and actions. Your need for control starts to fade, and your acceptance of everything becomes a natural reaction; you start to contemplate the deeper meaning of your existence, making your purpose your priority. Your individual identity starts blending into the universal oneness of unity, which reveals your higher Self-identity.

All lower expressions of the mind and thoughts become uninteresting and unattractive as a deep desire to live in the cosmic consciousness takes over. It's like being exposed to a genuine relationship of love through the highest form of expression. Once you

ROUTINE: THE KEY TO HEALTHY HABITS   41

experience this, all other lower expressions of love through lust, attachment, or fear become unworthy of your attention.

Your whole body and mind vibration changes when you keep practicing each day, and layers of ego importance drop aside and reveal the true aware Self. It's as if you are outside a door that you know is the gateway to your liberation. Once you know it is there, you can never go back to your normal life doing normal things for the sake of being normal.

Every person I have ever taught or guided onto the yogic path has been given one warning: "If you are planning lifelong routine changes where you will be challenged and tested continuously, but will live with great peace, purpose, and contentment, then this path is for you." If you go on this path nothing will stay the same, as all things will start to come into balance, and all people and things that are not in balance will leave your life. This is very attractive to many and frightening to others.

This path is for people who invite change and expect it continuously: we expect change, so there is no surprise at the unexpected. Our stability comes from keeping an open mind to uncertainties and what they will present. The old attitude of work hard, play hard, and then retire is not applicable any longer, especially to this modern and fast-paced life. The gap between young and old has become very narrow because of technology.

People are now not thinking about retiring as they see their lives as a whole and not in segments. This has actually prepared the younger generation for the mind-set to be more flexible and adaptable in their thinking and approach to life. If they have to find a new job or make new friends or move to a new environment, it's not a big deal. This is a great attribute to have because a yogi needs to be adaptable, adjustable, and accommodating in all situations and with all people. A yogi's mind cannot be rigid in its thinking or approach to life. Everything in and around us is ever changing and moving. Nothing is constant except inconsistency itself. Our minds need to get used to constant shifts because as one aspect of our life seems balanced, another aspect will need work or attention. This is the case for every soul on earth.

We have not taken the form of the body just to sit about and become comfortable. This is why our routine is of the utmost importance, so we never become too relaxed and lose our focus, consistency, and purpose.

Chapter Summary

- ◆ Make the way you live specific and not so open-ended. Don't be open to just anyone and anything that comes along.
- ◆ A routine is not to limit you, but to help you live with specific intentions and to support your goals.
- ◆ Respect the importance of setting healthy habits,

balance the boundaries of necessities, and lower the need for extras.

• Know every habit you form will make up some part of your daily routine and will either become a distraction or add to your life.

• Align your habits with nature and watch your physical and mental health become balanced.

• If in doubt, ask yourself if you really want to change a habit and if you are going to put in the effort. This way you will be consciously choosing change.

• Know exactly what you are filling your days with and why. This way you will be living the habits and routine you feel most connected with.

Daily Life Practices

There are many practices you can do to get started with a healthy routine, but the ones on the following pages are important and simple and will have the maximum effect as you begin creating new healthy habits.

The start to your day sets the tone for how you interact and communicate, but also affects your awareness and decisions you have to make. The close of your day is also important because you need to be conscious of all your actions, so if there are any that need adjusting, this would be the time to reflect on them and find a resolution.

PUTTING YOUR BEST FOOT FORWARD

Before you step out of bed, feel and sense from which nostril the air is flowing more freely.

Step out of bed with the foot that corresponds to the same side as the nostril that is flowing more freely. Now come up and stand on that foot and leg fully while balancing yourself on the ball of the opposite foot.

You are now standing straight on one leg and using the other foot's toes for balancing the body. Now breathe slowly and take seven breaths in and out through the nose.

This practice not only gets you to be conscious of the very first step you take out of bed to start your day but is also a yogic practice to align the energy of the mind and body with the earth and universal vibrations. As these opposing energies of positive and negative flow through the body, changing sides a few times ever hour, your energy level will be enhanced from the very first step you take in your day.

VOCAL ATTENTION

After flossing and brushing your teeth, scrape your tongue with a tongue scraper.

Then gargle with some premade sesame oil mixed with tea tree oil (in a ten-to-one ratio) through the teeth and around the mouth. Do this for a minute or two.

This practice will strengthen the gums and teeth and move excess mucus out of the throat. It's a great practice for making the voice sharp as you look to your day of speaking and communicating.

CLEANSING THE GATEWAY TO THE MIND FOR GREATER FOCUS

There are different ways to do this practice. The simplest is to use a neti pot to clean out the nasal cavity of all the excess mucus that has collected from the night's sleep.

Fill your neti pot up with warm water and add a few pinches of salt.

Wash out each nostril once or twice depending on the level of blockage. If you don't have a neti pot, cup your hand and add a little warm water and a tiny bit of salt. Sniff this into one nostril and spit the water out of your mouth. Repeat this on the other side.

REFLECTION AND CLOSURE

Sit and reflect on your day for thirty minutes to an hour before bed. Make sure to do this before you are sleepy. You need an alert mind for this practice.

What was an action or word you could have changed to make a conversation or communication move smoother? Did you attract what you wanted, or are you attracting people and work you are not energized about? What could you have done better? What needs to change in your attitude or actions to make things go peacefully? This practice is about what changes you can bring to your own actions and not anyone else's. Once you have identified one thing, make sure to take it into your day tomorrow and apply it.

Let your thoughts now slow down, and know tomorrow is the day when you take better actions, but now it is time for sleep. Prepare yourself for bed.

This practice is important for two reasons: first, because tomorrow you will be able to act with awareness and not continue doing something that is not getting you the desired results you are seeking. Second, many of our dreams are reflections on unresolved thoughts from our day, and we don't want to carry these into our sleep, thinking about how we should have acted differently. This practice allows us to find a resolution before we sleep so our mind can rest and not be filled with unnecessary stress.

Practice: The Key to Your Foundation

I could tell you an epic story of a great guru or sage from the Himalayas to illustrate the transformational power of spiritual practice, but that isn't necessary. And much of what happens is either unbelievable or so subtle that the mind has a hard time connecting it to the supernatural.

I know plenty of stories that are relevant to you and can bring home the same message and inspiration. These are stories from my clients and people who live now in our culture, in our everyday world; they have been doing their practice for years, living in joy and plugged into the universal energy called pure love.

The story of Jaimyse, my wife, is probably the best choice here. My wife and I don't have such dissimilar life stories, as she was working in the entertainment world as a young actress in TV commercials from the age of nine, then living the Hollywood life by marrying a movie star at the age of twenty.

Life was one big VIP lifestyle of private planes and living

in Paris while traveling the world. When I met her, she was living between New York and Los Angeles and running a theater company. Her life was somewhat quieter than it had been, but she frequently got ill and took a lot of medication, including antibiotics.

For a year or so she was my client and student; I treated her for bronchitis and other immune system issues, teaching her different morning practices in order for her to develop a personal practice. She was a quick learner and wanted to apply more to her life. After a while, she asked me if she could study with my guru in India. I organized this for her, and she went off for a few months to study.

During her "honeymoon" stage of learning in India, she felt amazing, especially as things were new and exciting. But isn't this the case when we discover new things? The real test comes when the romance of something new ends and we need to apply the teachings to "real life," bringing with it many conflicts, as the mind is resistant to change. These are the times either the mind surrenders to the higher Self or the ego fights hard to stay in its old habits.

I had humorously warned Jaimyse at the end of our first consultation that if she started to do a daily practice, take that first step on the yogic path, her life would not be the same anymore. Now she was finding this out for herself.

Often life becomes even more challenging when we first take

up a spiritual practice. This is the step before the mind realizes life has more meaning and joy, when it lets go of control. This is because spiritual practice expands our consciousness and brings awareness beyond what we are normally used to. But once this expansion starts, it begins to move and shift people and things in our life that are not vibrating at the same level.

Water seeks its own level because this is the law of nature. Spirituality follows the same law. Jaimyse was coming to many crossroads of understanding herself, living that truth and seeking her own level beyond the ordinary. This is a great leap of faith, to let go of what you know and to dive into the unknown. This is what a true seeker does.

I didn't see Jaimyse again for a couple of years before we met in Los Angeles to have lunch with a mutual friend visiting from India. I could tell something was very different about her now, but I didn't need to ask, because I knew she had been doing her yogic practices and living this lifestyle. There is a glow of inner beauty that shines from inside of people who know the value of practice and make it a part of their life. You can see it in their eyes—they become luminous.

Jaimyse had now taken the first steps to becoming a yogini, a female yogi, and was not just doing her daily practices but was in teacher training with another yogi and studying in India regularly every year. She was a single woman starting to focus on her purpose and spiritual life. She had taken the little I had given her and made it into a whole new life. This is the power of daily practice.

Now all that was left was to marry her.

The Practice of Mind Management

Sadhana is the repetition of our spiritual practice on a daily basis, over and over throughout our lifetime, and for a yogi over many lifetimes. I say *lifetimes* because yogis know the spirit lives on in other forms once its purpose here on earth is done. This is what makes us spiritual—we have a spirit that is our guide, which is why we refer to it as the higher Self or higher consciousness. It is not a person but pure energy that runs through our bodies and has its home in the heart chakra, or energy center, in the middle of the chest.

Our goal as yogis is to listen to and be guided by this energy, which communicates to our mind when necessary. It is guiding us through absolutely every aspect, event, and situation in our life, although we (the mind) might not be listening. That is why it is our guru and guide within and holds the power of the whole universe within it. It is the limitless and endless power that we are connected to. It's not the power of the mind, but the power and source that the mind pulls from. Then what is the mind?

When you say "me," "I," or "myself," who is this "me" or "I" that you are speaking about? It is the mind, or intellect. There is the mind at a lower level, and then spirit is the source at a higher, elevated level. They are sharing the same body.

The spirit is the energy that keeps the mind alive. It's the energy as well as the force behind our existence. The mind would not exist without the energy of the spirit. The mind rebels against this situation, because it likes to think of itself as an individual and separate from everything. It's like the child who wants to be independent, but at the same time knows she needs her home and parents. This is where all our problems have their root. A separate mind believes it has power, when actually it has little power of its own.

But the truth is that we need the mind, and it needs managing. Swami Niranjanananda said: "The highest spiritual practice in life is mind management. The highest awareness is how the mind responds to situations." He is speaking about the most important aspect of the yogic path, which is to control the mind. Without being able to control the mind (ourselves), there is no controlling our life, our actions, our habits, or our thoughts.

So how do you control your mind? This is a two-step process:

1. Learning and doing a daily spiritual practice.
2. Surrendering to the higher Self once the mind is calm.

But what do we know about the mind?

Modern science and yogic science differ in the way they view the mind. Here is how we look at the mind as yogis. The mind has four major parts, and these parts are the aspects and functions of the mind that work together to create thoughts, ideas, opinions, memories, etc. Let's go through these so you better understand why you think the way you do, and how to change thought patterns to more beneficial, kind, and joyful ones.

The first aspect of the mind is intellect. This is the higher mind aspect of the four parts. It is the power of discrimination but also analyzing and deducting to reach conclusions. When the intellect is balanced and receiving true knowledge from the other parts of the brain, it is in harmony with all beings and nature itself. Here we have an understanding that we are a part of a bigger sum total of humanity, all beings, and spirituality.

But when the intellect has too much theoretical information and has little experience of what it believes, it becomes imbalanced with all the theory it has collected. Here it starts to become a theoretical mind. Theory without action and personal experience leaves the intellect making up stories for itself. This creates static energy in the mind, because when you only inspect and analyze something, it doesn't mean you actually know it from life experience.

Our society has put a lot of emphasis on this aspect of the mind by inventing and creating so much stuff we have no use for, but we still continue to make and demand. We just come up with an intellectual reason why it is necessary and then market its desirability and value to our intellectual senses. A yogic definition of intelligence is very different; we don't consider someone as intelligent if they can design, build, and manufacture things that are not necessary for our collective existence. This is a waste of precious time. We see an intelligent person as one who has full control of the mind and therefore of themselves, as one who is living the purpose of their existence and not the purpose of their desires.

The next part of the mind is identity, or, as we have come to know it, the ego aspect of the mind. This is the part of the mind that identifies with things and influences the intellect. It is the aspect of the mind that has an agenda and wants to be heard, casting shadows on the higher mind. For example, it makes the intellect think the body needs to be a certain shape, so the intellect then tries to "get into shape." Or it brings up an old memory or emotion, which can take over and control your mind and actions. This is the aspect of the mind that creates confusion for itself.

The next aspect and function of the mind is the processor. This part of the mind processes the outside world and all the stimulation, communications, and interactions you are having and passes them on to the other parts of the mind, eventually landing in your memory bank. This part of the mind is just a process, and not an influencer or judge of what is happening. It doesn't know good or bad, but because the memory bank also feeds information from the past to the processor, it now has something to throw back out into the world.

The next and last part and function of the mind is the memory bank. This is the aspect of the mind that has a lot of influence over our thoughts, as it is constantly being fed more and more information to store. This memory bank also permeates the body through feeling and emotions. As you think, you become. Your mind is one big memory bank of past, present, and future thoughts. Everything you touch, taste, smell, see, and hear creates a memory through the processor of the mind, and is now stored in this part of the brain.

Most of our thoughts have some aspect of the past in them. As this is the most influential aspect of our mind, we are mostly living in the past, while being in the present and thinking of the future. Do you see your issue here? You are trying to stay in the moment, knowing it is the only real thing, but every sense memory is catapulting you into the past, while you plan the future, passing or missing the present brief moment. It is very popular for people to speak about being in the present and enjoying the moment, but few of us can actually do this.

We only know the past, because we have experienced it. All else is fiction yet to be lived. But at the same time, the past is not real anymore, as only the present is real. And the aspirations of the future (anytime from now to infinity) create fear of and excitement for the unknown. So the mind tricks itself.

Can you now understand the challenge in trying to stay and live in the moment? Do you see how the mind works against itself and can't be present because it is being fed and pulled by the different parts, which have their own agendas? The mind is like four coworkers with different job titles: the identity ego thinks it is the most important, the intellect is busy trying to work things out, the processor is too busy handling information, and the memory bank can't get enough to eat from the processor. It's chaos in this office!

You are creating your reality based on what is in the different parts of your mind, thoughts, and memory. This is only your reality and not anyone else's, which is why much of the time you may feel unheard, unloved, and misunderstood.

Do you now see why your only hope of escaping your chaotic mind is daily spiritual practice?

Now just sit for a moment and read though the last few paragraphs, because I really want you to understand what your mind is up against, and why having a practice is the answer to all your problems in life. I'm making a huge statement here, and you will one day look back after committing to this practice and understand its full meaning when you are living with clarity, joy, and a life purpose. This is not just my promise, it's your soon-to-be reality if you choose it.

This mess of a mind is the exact reason the yogis devised a spiritual practice, because they knew this was going to be the dilemma of human beings in this age. Ancient teachings from thousands of years ago speak about these times when the human mind will be confused with outside distractions, which the mind itself will create. Do you recognize the distractions and confusion around you? People are at war over the color of their skin, their sexual preference, their gender. Others are at war over religion, power, and economic gain. Some are at war over words, hurt feelings, or being rejected. And most people are at war in their own mind, beating themselves up for not being good enough, while others are pumping up their ego, thinking they are better than everyone. Do you recognize the chaos and misperception we are living? This is all a result of our collective thinking.

One who is lost can't lead others out of confusion. This is why we need to plug in each day through our practice and be fed by the source of all creation. Otherwise we stay in our delusions, which have become our reality. And nothing about this process is theoretical. Yogic life and spiritual practice are a scientific and practical way of grinding the mind into submission so the real boss can take over. The process is about learning the practices and then doing them every day. It's that simple. And by doing them, you experience their fruits.

As you practice, Mother Nature and the universal energy will support you in the process, because you are moving away from the mind exerting control over your actions and instead being guided by this energy. It becomes a team effort, so to speak, in which you are not alone but have the most powerful vibration as your partner in life.

The Steps to Transcendence

The yogi can answer the ultimate question of why you are and what is your purpose with: do your sadhana, your spiritual practice, every day, and the answers will come. There is no one in the world who can answer this question for another. There is an answer; it just needs to come from within yourself, and the way of extracting it is practice.

This is the part of life no one else can do for you. It's the key to unlocking the biggest and deepest questions we need answered. It is a journey we must make alone, but not in a solitary manner. We are always traveling with the source of creation and at times with other souls too. It's not that other people can't join in your life, or you can't share in their lives, but the actual practice needs to be done alone. It's between you and the higher divine Self who guides you into deeper knowledge. The teacher of all teachers, the yogi within you, is the one you want to be listening to, becoming, and reflecting on the outside.

I know this goes somewhat against doing your practice in groups and in studios, but your personal practice is about listening, surrendering, and doing in silence that which is not possible in outer surroundings with lots of people and distractions. So you should always do your practice in the morning alone, and then join groups and classes as an extra gathering for chanting and *satsang*, which is Sanskrit for a spiritual discourse or sacred gathering. Otherwise you will never get that enlightenment you are seeking.

The first level of sadhana is to balance the body through flexibility and movement, helping to remove stiffness and stagnant energy. This is what people know as *asana* or postures. At this level you are being cleansed of toxins from inside by moving your body into different shapes while twisting, bending, and inverting. This level of practice has become the one most people identify with in yoga, because it is physical. Our world is very physical, so it is no surprise that this physical level gets more attention than all the other aspects of yoga, which are much more subtle. But this physical level has its limits and is the least important of the practices. It is a level that if focused on for too long will lead to its own kind of stagnation of energy, because it was only designed to be an optional step before moving on to breathing practices.

As you move into breathing and concentration, or meditation practices, layers of mental and emotional blocks that have been stifling the mind and not allowing you to live in a limitless manner will be cleared. At this level, you are cleansing the subtle channels of deep-seated toxins and subtle energy blockages.

At the beginning stages, the practices will start to balance these levels and you will experience an ease of body and mind. This is already a great stage of achievement to reach if it is your goal to be more peaceful and calm, and to live with balance of health. As we practice more and over many years, we start to elevate into higher and expansive levels of consciousness that become known only to those who are disciplined and diligently practice daily.

It's similar to a walk through the hills: when it seems like you have reached your destination and you approach the top of the hill, you then see the top of the next hill before you. This yogic journey is like that. That's why it needs work, and you need to make it important enough to be able to advance forward, remembering that it is a journey without an end, but one you will live fully. But just like the walk through the hills, this journey is full of rivers, forests, wild animals, and many other adventures, so you never become lazy or bored unless you stop walking.

As long as you make the effort to keep moving forward, there is so much to see and experience. You will feel such serenity and love for nature and all beings that when you get back to your normal day-to-day life you will want to share this feeling with everyone else. This is the effect of pure sadhana. It makes you feel universal and not just worldly.

It's time to feel universal.

A Thought Diet

In these times of science and intellectualism, being clever and smart is determined by how much information and knowledge

a person has collected and how much of it they can repeat. If
the mind has a photographic memory, then the person will even
be labeled as a genius. If we make a "smart" device, then we are
creative. If we are a great public speaker, we are charismatic. If we
invent stuff, we are amazing. If we build a profitable company, we
are savvy. The labels are endless.

At school we are taught to be clever by passing our exams, no
matter how we accomplish the goal—by studying or by memo-
rizing. In business, we are expected to make lots of money to be
a success. These are signs that we are putting our mind to good
use. The popular belief says that to be clever or smart we need
to be informed. This is the same notion that teaches that if we
ask more questions, we will have more answers. But we know
from experience that asking one too many questions starts to
make the mind confused as it compares information with other
information. This process, as I mentioned before, will produce
doubt in our mind, and a doubtful mind is an indecisive one.
It's one that is not sure of the truth. It's also a mind that can be
overwhelmed and controlled easily by another mind. The mind
needs a master, and if it is not the higher Self it will be someone
else's mind.

Knowledge and information are different sides of the same
coin. Information is turned into knowledge when we put it into
practice, and the result of practice is experience. So it is a step-by-
step process. Information is something we may collect and repeat,

but it never turns into knowledge (knowing) if we don't put the information into practice. If a person has heard of an elevator but has never seen or used one, they may have some information about it moving up and down, but they will not have the proper knowledge about how it feels. Their information is theoretical and lacking experience. Once they have the experience of riding in an elevator, then all the information they had before becomes replaced by the actual experience itself.

From an early age we are told to ask, advance, compete, and collect, but not much is taught to us about the dilemma of having too much on our mind and thinking too much. Ask anyone around you and pretty much everyone will say they can't stop thinking— even for a second. People are now medicating in various ways just so they can slow their minds down, so the thoughts can travel fifty miles per hour instead of their normal hundred miles per hour. We are in real need of the "consciousness police" to pull us over and send us to the Zen traffic school to slow down.

As I work with so many people and get to know about their daily routines and habits, I see more clearly how our society is functioning. I rarely hear the habits of stillness and silence spoken about. In a world of excess and information overload, stillness and silence should be the tools of choice not just to block out noise but to understand what information to take in and what to leave out.

In silence there is clarity. In noise there is confusion.

In stillness there is calm. In excess motion there is excess nervous energy.

I experience at least two hours of stillness and silence throughout my day, as these are the moments I can observe my thoughts. A minute here and a minute there can really allow the mind to rest, and I practice this all day. Between sending emails, speaking on the phone, cooking, and working, I make sure to be in silence and stillness enough of the time to bring about balance. But some days are very challenging when things get busy. This is when I practice a little more often to keep my balance.

Hoarding is hoarding—and not just as it pertains to material objects. Thoughts are also "things" and can be hoarded. How many times have the same thoughts looped through your mind, and you just don't know how to let them go? The mind is hoarding thoughts that we are fearful of letting go: maybe thoughts of an old relationship, what your next meal will be, or the morning's conversation. It is all in the memory of the mind, being played over and over again like a broken record.

To go on a thought diet is not to stop thinking altogether but to slow down the thinking enough for the mind to feel peaceful. It's also about thinking more quality thoughts and less quantity of thoughts. It's turning your focus from fact gathering to bringing your attention to the things that have importance. It's being much more specific and selective about what you think about or expose the senses to.

Imagine your house is on fire and you have time to grab a few things. You're not likely to head to the trash and take the trash out. You are going to get all living beings and valuables out first. You are going to focus on the important things and forget about the unimportant things. This approach is how you are going to focus on the essential thoughts and discard the remainder.

Losing Those Mental Pounds

To lose those extra mental pounds we need to do two things. First, we have to use and edit the information we already have. This way the mind and memory are not collecting new information to store that is in conflict with the information you already have. When I see the news, I never think this information is the truth. I just treat it as part truth, part information, and part entertainment. This way I forget it quickly from my immediate awareness and don't accept it or repeat it. It's in the repeating and thinking about it that it becomes a stronger part of your memory. This is also because this news is constantly changing and morphing into more news and more endless stories. So knowing the story will keep evolving and expanding, I catch just a few bits of it but never the entirety, enough for it to bother my mind.

Second, as we slow down the collection of new information, we must start to become very selective about what we let into our brain.

This means to be selective about what conversations we have, what we speak about, and with whom we hang out. It's editing the different environments we pass through, exercising discrimination when watching something. For example, while writing this I am sitting at a communal table at a coffee shop with multiple people chatting away around me. People are speaking next to me, but I am only picking up a word or two they are saying because my focus is on writing.

I know that I can write and not be disturbed by people in this particular environment because there is plenty of natural light, fresh air, and light background music. I can stay focused. Now if I were to try and write in a bar with music and drinking around me or in a place where I had a lot of friends who wanted to chat, I would have no hope of focusing. So I avoid those people and situations when I need to focus on something important to me. This is a simple example of using discrimination, so the mind can stay focused and not take on more noise, distractions, and information.

Avoiding Excesses and Extremes

When you avoid excesses and extremes, you will get a good grip on controlling the senses. The mentality of living our life to the fullest usually means to live the highs and lows. No one really wants to live the lows, but they are a natural outcome of many highs. If you climb the highest mountains in the world, they have extreme weather conditions and altitudes that the body and mind have to suffer through.

Then as you descend you will feel the effects of the altitude drop, which creates another round of extreme pressure on your system. In the same way, if you eat until you are full, it is an extreme for the body and mind to deal with. If you do this once it has a less negative outcome, but if you do it most of your life it has more serious consequences.

Thus the highs and lows give the body and mind all their ailments and pain. But most people who hear this reasoning ask, "Isn't life boring without the ups and downs, the highs and lows, or the emotional thrills?" It all depends on what the purpose and intention of your life is. If you are looking to go with the flow and experiment with your body and mind, then the highs and lows will be a natural reaction to this way of living. If you feel that this makes your life more interesting, then this is how you should live. But this doesn't lead to the balanced life that a yogi strives to live.

If you want to live in balance with your body and mind, then you won't experience anything that is an extreme. When you get to the point where the body or mind seems to be tipping the scale and becoming irritated, agitated, very excited, or too energetic, you will recognize the extreme and pull back a little to the point of balance, which is the focal point of the yogic life.

Your Nature

Understanding your basic nature will help you understand why you behave the way you do. This holds the key to why you push your senses to the point of extremes and become out of control. From birth you have a certain characteristic that is particular to you, and it stays a part of your life until your last breath. This becomes our nature that affects everything we do and all the decisions we make.

It's karma in action, it affects karma, and it is karma itself.

When observing a child we can identify characteristics that suggest what kind of an adult they are going to grow into. Particular mannerisms tell you what kind of human they will be and how they will act. Just ask a mother or father. They will describe their children twenty years in the future. Either we have the extreme in us or we don't. Of course, circumstances also influence our behavior patterns, and so do the experiences we have been through, but our natural character from birth will either make those patterns more extreme or not. For instance, my nature from childhood has not been very extreme. So when there were opportunities in my life to take more, eat more, buy more, or talk more, I usually leaned toward being less extreme. This was also so I didn't feel out of control. This has been my nature since I was a child. There are times when I have behaved out of character because of my environment or the influence of others around me, but I have always come back to my basic nature, which seeks quiet and solitude. And this is still true today.

For us to start taking control of the senses and taming them, we will need to modify and shift our habits so they are not causing the senses to be out of balance in the first place. If we are successful at this shift, we will still need to deal with the outside world, which also has its own nature. Mother Nature has her own natural shifts through the seasons and weather patterns that have an effect on us. Other people around us have their own particular nature and energy that affect us.

Every single environment we enter is interacting with our energy and mind. Now take all these combinations of people, places, and energies and put them all together and you should be able to get a sense of why we have all the issues we do, not just in society but in our bodies and minds.

We are so overloaded with information and stimulation that just hearing a song, a voice, or a sentence can set us off into a panic or stressed emotional state. As individuals and as a society, we have become so sensitive to words, foods, and other stimulation that our health is suffering for it. We need to have practices we can lean on to help our senses and emotions become silent and more balanced. These practices don't need to be so complicated, but need to be practiced regularly as a part of our lifestyle and yogic mind-set.

Following the yogic teachings helps us also to have fewer desires and to think more of the collective community called earth/humanity. As this helps to lower our outer self-importance and tame our ego identity, we will start to have thoughts and ideas that are good for Mother Nature, that don't pollute, and that don't have a destructive or negative effect on our nervous system.

Yogis always edit what they take in through the eyes, ears, skin, nose, and mouth. Every single sensory interaction or energy, be it a cell phone or food, has either a negative, destructive effect or a healing and cleansing effect on us and the earth. We just have to choose well and edit a lot out so we are not overloading our senses—keeping a balance in an unbalanced world is our challenge as yogis.

Breath and the Science of Your Life Force

Have you tried to stop breathing lately? An odd question, you might think! Maybe you haven't tried to stop breathing on purpose, but had to as a reaction to immense fear or something that was just so amazing it took your breath away. It's an intense but mostly terrifying feeling when we think we can't breathe or are frantically gasping for air.

Just the other day, I was eating a piece of fruit that got stuck in my throat and I couldn't breathe. It seemed that time had stopped. I went into stillness for a moment, because I know freaking out makes the situation much worse. The key was to avoid trying to breathe, and at the same time, work out the solution to the problem with calmness.

Looking back at the experience of choking, when my mind decided to stay still and listen to what was the answer, my actions happened instinctively. I didn't actually do any thinking as such. Intuition, the inner voice, just guided my hands and actions before the process of fear and thinking could take control. This is the power of stillness. Through stillness and silence the mind is calm and the inner voice takes over.

Was this a bad experience? Not at all. It was needed so I could practice trust and stillness, silence, and listening, and ultimately work through a potential fear in the memory bank. This memory will now serve me well for another time of potential fear or danger.

What is unknown and a hidden mystery is that the breath operates on many deeper levels, performing functions that are simply miraculous and very powerful. It is a great force that is unseen by the eyes but felt in every part of our being. It's the silent energy that on a physical level keeps us alive. But on the subtle level, this energy allows us to communicate and travel beyond our body or mind into the spiritual realm using all our chakras and other energy points. In other words, the breath is not just the power of the divine but is the divine in motion because it contains prana. Prana is not the breath itself, but it is the subtle energy of the breath that gives it power. It is the actual life force of the body and mind.

A yogi understands how to maneuver and use this life force according to the ancient teachings, through the use of yogic practices and rituals. This is how the power of prana reveals itself in every aspect of life through the body and mind. There is a whole science behind our breath and prana. Every element has a heavier and more subtler force behind it that performs functions on many levels. Just as fire is the physical manifestation of friction and heat, our breath is the physical part of prana that keeps the body working.

Prana, the vital life force, moves about in our body in five different ways:

1. *Prana*: the breath entering the system
2. *Apana*: moves down in the body
3. *Samana*: moves inward toward the center of the body
4. *Vayana*: moves outward toward the outer surface of the body
5. *Udana*: moves upward in the body

It is the movement of these five energies, like a perfectly executed dance routine, that allows our body and mind to function immaculately. It is through the subtle movement of this pranic energy that every organ operates and functions. Therefore, every aspect of our well-being depends on the correct use of this force. Hence the term *pranayama*—the control and directing of our breath and life force. This is why in ayurvedic medicine it is considered that *vata,* or the element of air that is the cause of all movement in the body, is the main cause of all nervous disorders and the majority of health issues. In the body air is constantly in movement as the blood is circulating, the heart is pumping, or toxins are exiting. This is all a function of our breath and prana. When the five pranas are not flowing in the right direction or in the correct amount, we consider this the beginning of all diseases.

Prana is also food and nourishment to the bodily systems. It feeds them vital energy. The sun, moon, air, food, and rain all provide prana to us and the earth, which is one big breathing pranic organism. The earth is constantly feeding and cleaning itself, as is our body. And all these functions are happening through and affected by our breathing habits. When we speak about pollution, we are referring to the fact that the earth and our bodies can't breathe properly and fully.

Prana and Breathing Patterns

Our life expectancy is directly connected to the use of our breath. The yogis say that we come into the world with a certain amount of breaths, and as slowly or quickly as we choose to use them up, life in the body will be longer or shorter. So the slower we breathe the longer life we can expect to live.

A normal person at rest takes between twelve and sixteen breaths per minute. These breaths are usually very shallow and quick. They are also always influenced by our activities, thoughts, and emotional state. Deep, slow breathing calms everything down, while quick breathing moves everything more rapidly. As yogis we want to bring the breathing down to five to seven breaths a minute during our normal activities, and one to three breaths during our practice in the morning. This is how the mind starts to be calm and still.

Modern society is constantly in the pursuit of more health and energy. We have been taught that if we drink caffeine or eat energy bars we can get more energy. But we are unaware that our body actually produces energy and possesses the most powerful energy through the use of prana. The mind has become programmed to believe that we have to consume something to get energy, not that we already have a storehouse of energy that we must learn how to use when needed. As I tell my clients, it's as if you are hungry and need money for food, and all the time you have a pocketful of money but never remember to use it.

When we practice deep, slow yogic breathing, we are increasing absorption of oxygen and energy in our entire system. Much of our fatigue and lack of energy comes from our *nadis,* or channels, that are blocked and unable to circulate energy and not from not having energy.

We have seventy-two thousand of these channels in our body that need to be kept open and circulating nourishment to all our systems. When respiration is slow, long, and deep, our food, drink, and even our thoughts are circulated to every part of our being through the nadis. This creates a flow that makes the body and mind function at optimal health. This is because there are no blockages being created and every part is receiving the energy it needs. When a person is not aware of their breath and is breathing shallower or at times even holding the breath unconsciously, some of these channels become blocked, impaired, or deficient. This blockage in the physical form is like excess cholesterol buildup in the arteries from the lack of prana to break it down, or in a more subtle form, like asthma or a headache through the channels not receiving enough prana.

The performance of the brain is also directly linked to the function and use of the breath. Prana provides the energy and food the brain needs to function on higher levels of consciousness. When the mind is still, prana flows correctly through the brain, giving it guidance beyond the ordinary ego level. This is when the thoughts are elevated beyond trying to fulfill our personal wants and desires and expand our awareness to include the entire world as a community. This is when we use our intellect power. It's when we feel the heartbeat of the earth as a living entity and connect to all living beings beyond just a human form. This is everyone's potential if they practice and live even a small part of the yogic path. But even if it is not your goal to reach the highest levels, by breathing correctly you will still be living in health, harmony, and much more awareness than what you normally experience.

Peace, purpose, and even-mindedness are what a yogi is striving for. In this state of mind we can go from thinking to just being. This is an even greater place to be than happiness, as happiness also has an extreme opposite, which is sadness. Both happiness and sadness become a distraction on the yogic path. This is why contentment is taught by great sages as a more balanced state of mind to be in. It is an even-minded state where there are fewer emotions and sensory distractions for our mind to be disturbed by. We are less likely to have emotional mood swings, highs and lows depending on a particular situation. Instead, we are balanced, which offers clarity of mind and actions. We don't react on an emotional whim but out of our contentment.

Committing to our breathing practices for longer periods during our morning practice will over time make a natural progression wherein yogic breathing will become the normal way of breathing for you during your day. In this way the body and mind will no longer be susceptible to everyday imbalances. Common behaviors like rushing, impatience, and reacting defensively that lead to deeper-seated thought patterns of ignorance, self-indulgence, and miscommunication start to shift out of our consciousness. The mind starts to become filled with a universal way of being. Our earth is suffering, and we are suffering with it. We are focused on building superpowers and not loving power. We don't think inclusively but exclusively, and for this we suffer.

Our breath is the connection between our body and mind

and to our fellow beings. One is an extension of the other. As we breathe in, we are nourishing our whole system and feeding the brain pranic energy. And when we breathe out, we are cleaning the body of toxins and unusable gases. This is why our body is a nourishing and cleaning machine all in one unit. For anyone who is looking to give their body the best nourishing energy along with the most comprehensive cleansing, pranayama is the technique they should use. It's a scientific way of doing things. There is no need to understand it beyond the basics. Just do it and you will find out for yourself. Become the scientist and experiment.

The breath is either a voluntary or involuntary physiological process. On one hand, if you don't pay any attention to the breath, it will happen automatically but unevenly and more shallowly. This has to do with people's habits and posture, as most people don't sit up properly to have an open chest. They also don't physically push out the stomach when inhaling. Many people do the reverse and suck in the stomach when inhaling, which is another reason for shallow breathing.

Breathing will also follow the rhythm of the mind and thoughts. But if you focus on it and take control through yogic methods, you can control all of the body's systems and make the breath voluntary. The nervous, circulatory, and cardiovascular systems, for example, are very quickly and quite easily controlled through the breath. This is breathing in a voluntary manner where we are conscious of our inhalation and exhalation, controlling the length and duration of each. When we breathe involuntarily, the breath is at the beck and call of the nervous system and senses. So when any emotions like excitement or fear come along, the breath follows suit and moves more rapidly and becomes out of balance. This is why we frequently experience being out of breath or find ourselves holding our breath unconsciously.

Ultimately we are doing these practices for two reasons. One is for our daily life and all that we will encounter in our personal twenty-four hours, so we can come out of our day with more peace and health. The second and main point is for us to be able to elevate to greater heights in our spiritual practice and stay plugged into that energy all day. Every morning I connect with the universal force, and it slowly wears off during the day until I sleep and connect again the next morning. It's just how my electric car works!

So now you have some theoretical knowledge of what to expect from our practice and your yogic journey. Now it is time to start learning how to do a proper sequence of these practices so you can also have the practical experience. This is where the yogi becomes the scientist.

The Yogi Code Practices

The daily Yogi Code Practices I introduce in this section provide the foundation and support for the rest of your day as well as for reaching the goals of each chapter. These five morning practices help you feel grounded and fully supported on the physical, mental, and spiritual levels. Once you have integrated this foundation as part of your routine, you will be ready to add new practices and exercises that appear at the end of each chapter in the section called "Daily Life Practices."

You will notice that I have not added asana (yoga postures) in this sequence. Asana is a good practice to open up the body and make it more flexible, but it is not a necessary part of a spiritual practice. If you have a favorite posture practice, then do that before these practices below. You can also find videos on asana sequences and all the other practices I outline on YCMembership.com.

At the end of the book, I provide a "Twenty-One-Day Yogi Code Kick-Start" so you can kick-start your practice as well as become familiar with many more of the practices from the other chapters. This way you will have a great beginning to your practice and be able to stay enthusiastic and committed every day.

THE FULL YOGIC BREATH

No matter how much I write about pranayama and spiritual practices, the full yogic breath will always be the first one I discuss. It is the beginning and end of all breathing practices insomuch as it is a complete practice on its own. If you don't do any other practice, do this one.

When I teach this practice, I tell people to do it not only in the morning but during the whole day. If they encounter a stressful person or situation, for example, they can use it to calm the mind and avoid a conflict. I challenge anyone to do this breathing technique and try to become emotional. It isn't possible. When prana is flowing so perfectly and correctly, nothing can bother you. It has literally saved my life a few times, including the time I almost choked, as I mentioned earlier.

Before undertaking other more advanced breathing practices, we have to make sure we are breathing in and out fully and correctly, meaning that we are using the full capacity of the lungs. As most people breathe in a very shallow or interrupted manner, doing this practice sets the rhythm for all the other practices to come.

Shallow breathing is the cause of many physical aliments like bad circulation, heart weakness, and blood pressure issues, but the main illnesses are really the psychological ones like anxiety and depression. These mental disorders occur due to the improper gas exchange on the physical level and lack of prana on the subtle plane. It's like you have a huge capacity for energy and vitality but you are managing with much less.

The lungs are like balloons that fill up to the extent that we use them by inhaling and exhaling properly. As people today breathe in a more shallow way, full breathing is now referred to as "deep breathing."

As we are not breathing in fully and don't use our maximum lung capacity, the body and mind miss out on nourishment of the blood and energizing our system. And as we don't exhale fully, some carbon dioxide and other impurities remain and slowly start to poison the blood. Breathing correctly is more powerful than any food, medicine, or treatment you could ever have. This is why some yogis live only on prana and never eat or drink anything. Learn to do these practices and you will conquer many of your health issues as well as start to live with an amazing amount of energy.

From my experience with students in workshops, not many people know how to fully breathe properly. And most yoga practitioners think this is a basic practice and tend to overlook it, favoring more complicated practices. Full yogic breathing is a simple practice but one that will take a lifetime to master.

CONTROL OF THE SENSES

Controlling our senses is one of the most challenging aspects of the yogic path. From a young age we learn that life should be about having fun, seeking pleasure, and making things happen. Because of this belief system, as kids and into adulthood, most people strive to live up to this life goal. Part of having a good time is enjoyments and pleasures. The forms of enjoyments are many and varied, but there are a few main ones: entertainment, comfort, and relaxation.

Through entertainment, comfort, and relaxation, we have invented all kinds of material objects to amuse us and satisfy our desire for pleasure. But dedicating our lives to the pursuit of fun and relaxation has become our weakness. Haven't you noticed anytime you board a plane or enter an office or a home, someone is bound to say, "sit down and relax"?

Of course, while we manage to have these wants and enjoyments in place, all is fine and our senses are very satisfied or overloaded through stimulation. But when we don't get something we want, our mood takes a sudden downturn and we feel out of control. Like a child whose toy has been taken away, our mind starts to go through withdrawal and unhappiness. Losing a comfort or pleasure that we've come to depend on is a shock to the mind. It easily can cause depression, anxiety, and anger. I've seen people stress about not being able to relax. It's a strange dilemma to have.

If we look at what has really happened at the root level, we find our senses have been disturbed. Without the senses there is no enjoyment or need for comfort or relaxation. It is sensory perception and action that allows us to feel. And like an amplifier, our senses can amplify our experiences, which happens because of the intensity with which we do something. For instance, if you eat one meal a day, the sense of taste will be less stimulated and attached to food than if you eat five meals a day, making your palate oversaturated and numb to tastes. If you speak for most of the day, the sense of hearing and speech will be more sensitive to noise than if you talk for only half the day. Our senses are just reacting to the amount of sensory stimulation they are put through.

When you push too hard and move to the levels of extreme, the senses become overloaded and the body and mind try to protect themselves. This is when you start to get discomfort as a sign that you are pushing the system out of balance.

The way to control the senses is:

1. Through yogic practices included in this book.
2. Through mindfulness of your activities and maintaining balance through your actions and reactions.

While doing yogic practice is going to balance the mind and energize the body in the morning, we are not doing these practices all day. The main way you are going to control the mind is by not stimulating your senses too much. This is done through living a healthy, spiritual, and purposeful lifestyle, which is discussed in the following chapters.

CONCENTRATION AND MEDITATION

The mind is a muscle. It gets its exercise through thinking and contemplating things. It gets its rest by having fewer thoughts. And like a muscle it can become over- or underworked. At no time is the mind empty, as it is the nature of the mind to collect the information that the senses are reacting to and reflecting on. The mind is a storehouse, and the senses create its content. Even when the body is asleep, the mind is still busy because of the memory bank.

For all the patients and clients around the world whom I have treated or consulted with over the years, overstimulation of some sort is always the issue with their life. For example, I had a client named Jenny who came to me with issues related to migraines and skin rashes. I asked her to tell me about her daily routine. "What do you do first thing when you wake up?"

"I reach for my phone and check my messages, social media, and emails," she replied.

"Then what?" I asked.

She said she goes to the kitchen and makes coffee. Then she goes on her computer and reads the news. Then she usually makes a fruit shake or green juice or eats some yogurt on granola with milk. Then she gets into her car and drives to work while listening to a talk show.

"What's the environment like at work?"

"Crazy, hectic, mad, and busy, but that's normal." Then she told me she eats her lunch at her desk while on the phone or computer.

"How do you get to work?" I asked.

"The train or car, depending on if I am rushed or not."

"So you take the car if you are rushed?"

"Yes," she replied. *Hope I'm not the driver in front of you on the highway,* I thought. I was going to ask her more questions, but I already knew the cause of her ailments: overstimulation of her senses and approach to life. Her mind was so stimulated beyond its boundaries of health and well-being that it was exhibiting symptoms like migraines and overheating the skin to form eczema.

I suggested this to her, and she replied, "But this is the way I have always been. And my work colleague is doing the same, and she's fine." This is a pretty standard answer I hear a lot. I was also thinking how much unnecessary information was passing through her mind. Overinformation and overstimulation. Not a good combination on the peaceful path.

Jenny was exercising her mind muscle in a very destructive, excessive, "normal" way that wasn't sustainable in the long run. At nineteen, you can cope with this elevated, stimulated level of energy even though you have some health issues, but imagine what it does to the system at forty.

Most people complain about thinking too much and not being able to switch it off. And yet they keep collecting more unneeded information through stimulation, which they just see as normal. These thoughts are like the weights in the gym. They vary in heft. Some weigh a lot and some are lighter. The more our thoughts are tied to our senses and emotions the heavier they become, and as we grow in awareness and move deeper in consciousness our thoughts become lighter. The lighter ones we forget quicker, but the heavier thoughts are the ones we repeat again and again, creating more heaviness for the brain to deal with.

Right now, become aware of something you repeated a few times in your mind or out loud to someone today. Was it true? Was it worthwhile? Was it peaceful? What was the result?

The popular belief has now become that to meditate all we have to do is sit quietly and close our eyes, or that we can be in a state of meditation simply by chanting a mantra. For anyone who has done this, you will have experienced that meditation is not a quick and easy process. This is why concentration (or we could say "mindfulness") is the step before meditation on the yogic path. We have misinterpreted a very powerful practice—meditation—and made it mainstream, when it is actually a very exclusive practice.

When I say *exclusive,* I am not using the word as understood by the ego to mean "to exclude," but in the sense that it is a process and practice that is exclusively reached after many other practices like the ones I have mentioned in this chapter. In other words, meditation is not a stand-alone practice, which is why most people who "meditate" become frustrated or give up after some time.

The frustration arises because it is unrealistic to think you can empty the mind or just forget everything and sit quietly without first preparing the mind through other practices. Do you expect to reach a far-off destination quickly without some sort of transportation? Do you expect a roomful of children who are excited about a birthday party to sit still and be quiet? So, logically speaking, how can the mind become motionless and without thoughts just by us sitting quietly? In the Zen Buddhist tradition, meditation is taught as a distinct practice. But they use methods like we do in the Vedic or yogic tradition, which calls it *dharana* or concentration. This is treated as a preparatory step before meditation.

As we discussed, the mind is many things: an observer, collector, and recorder. So to catch its attention we need one thing that interests it above all the rest—just one object, sound, or image that becomes its "object of concentration" so it can focus on that and let all else fade into the background. When the mind has become engrossed in just one thing, then it becomes controlled and quiet. It means that nothing else has the attention of the mind but that one sound, image, or object. Remember the times when the whole day went by and you didn't even know how it happened because you were focusing on a project? This is similar to that focus. It is one-pointed and uninterrupted.

One-pointed attention comes from having the correct practice.

It is not the practice that is powerful but the practicing that brings out the power. People often ask me for "powerful" or "secretive" practices like a sacred mantra. "Give me a mantra that is powerful," students ask me. Or, like Swami Niranjanananda was saying at one of his talks, "People come to me and say, 'Swamiji, give me higher practices. I know I am ready for them.'" In reality there are no higher or lower practices. There are no levels one, two, or three, or advanced or beginner. They are all the same, with the distinction that one is the beginning, and as the mind practices, the energy of that practice keeps expanding into something greater but not higher. In this case it is only through the repetition of the practice that the vibration elevates or becomes more intense and not because we start a higher practice.

I never consider the teachings I teach or the practices I do as advanced. I always consider that I am at the beginning doing basic practices and that I am not advancing or arriving at any higher level. This way my ego doesn't mistakenly feed the other parts of the mind false information that it has achieved or created or done anything. On the yogic path we (the mind) don't take credit for anything; otherwise we are under the false impression that we are important. This way all credit goes to the higher Self, and the mind is free of conflict with itself and the world outside. With this attitude the mind is under control.

Chapter Summary

- Be patient with your practice. Don't expect to be a master while being an apprentice. Know your level and focus on doing the practices correctly.
- Do the practice daily. The key to progress is consistency, not how much time you practice.
- Make practice a priority, more important than anything else you do during that time. This way you won't be distracted before you have finished.

* Do your best but have no expectations. Expectations are a distraction on the yogic path.
* Have great respect for your spiritual practice and treat it as a blessing and a lifeline.

Your Yogi Code Practice

PREPARING YOUR PLACE OF PRACTICE

You should ideally always use the same spot for your spiritual practice, because that area starts to vibrate with your energy and the energy you are creating through your practice. It is also beneficial to have some tools that you use to help calm the mind and prepare it for the practice.

Two things I recommend you use are incense and tamboura sound. Incense such as sandalwood helps to calm the sense of smell and bring in a scent, which is transformative for the mind to become more inward and focused. Tamboura, also known as a tanpura, is an Indian drone instrument that makes a sound that harmonizes the vibration of the mind, helping it concentrate and focus more easily. You can find a tamboura track on YCMembership.com.

Before beginning, make time to set the intention for your practice. Why are you doing your practice? What do you want from your practice? What will you do with the great effects and energy produced by your practice?

Be specific and not open-ended so the soul/spirit/universe can guide you where you intend to go.

If you are not sure what you need or want, then just ask that your practice bring you clarity as to what the higher Self wants your mind to do today. This way you will be living your divine purpose.

STARTING YOUR PRACTICE

Here is how your daily Yogi Code Practice should be done at home. This practice should be the first thing you do after brushing your teeth and bathing.

You can either prepare the body with some asana postures if you already have a sequence you do regularly, find specific sequences on YCMembership.com, or go straight into your breathing practices.

Keep the eyes closed during these practices unless otherwise instructed. Having the eyes closed will help you go further inward. Always breathe through the nose if possible. (You will be able to see a demonstration of these practices on YCMembership.com.)

Full Yogic Breath
  • Sit on the floor in a cross-legged position (if your knees are off the floor, sit on a hard, solid cushion or blankets

until your knees are farther down than your hips) or sit
on a chair with your spine straight.

- Start to inhale, first feeling the stomach expand
  outward, then the rib cage, and then the chest, in this
  order. When exhaling, first feel the chest deflate, then
  the rib cage, and finally the stomach. Don't force the
  air out by pushing, but rather control the air by letting
  it out slowly. To exhale fully, pull the stomach in all the
  way without straining until all the air has been exhaled
  from the lungs.
- Inhale again, expanding stomach, rib cage, and chest.
  Exhale, deflating the chest, rib cage, and stomach,
  which is pulled in all the way.
- Make the breath very controlled, slow, and deep so at
  no time do you force the air in or out quickly and lose
  control over it.
- Do this practice for three to seven minutes or seven to
  fifteen rounds.
- Sit quietly for a moment and see how the practice
  affects your mind.

Humming Bee (*Bhramari*)
This practice involves the closing off of our senses so we can experience what it is like when our mind is not influenced by them. As
you will see, the mind will start to be filled with more peace and

fewer preoccupations. The special part of the practice is a humming noise, which vibrates in the ears, mouth, eyes, and nose and
is calming to the mind. It can also bring emotions to the surface,
but in a quiet and controlled way.

- To start the practice, sit in a comfortable seated posture
  so you are very stable and your back is straight.
- Now bring your arms up, open the elbows outward,
  and put your index finger into your ears. Don't press
  your fingers in too hard, but also not too lightly.
- Keep the mouth and lips closed, with the teeth
  slightly apart. Inhale very slowly through the nostrils.
  Exhale through the nose while making a long, even,
  and steady humming noise. Don't force the breath,
  but do it smoothly. Rest your arms between each
  round if they become tired; otherwise, do the rounds
  consecutively.
- Do five rounds.
- Sit quietly for a moment and see how the practice
  affects your mind.

Chakra Purification Focus (*Unmani Mudra*)

Chakras are energy centers running up and down our spine that
hold and distribute immense energy. They are also centers that
need maintenance in order to be ready for one of the most pow-

erful forces, called Kundalini, to go through them. This force is dormant at the base of the spine and needs awakening through yogic practice. In this practice we are stimulating the chakras and preparing them for this energy rise.

- Sit in a comfortable seated posture with a straight spine.
- Bring your attention to the back of your head at the top of the spine. Inhale and hold the breath for a second. Exhale slowly in a controlled manner, letting the air out very slowly. As you exhale, visualize your energy descending through the spine (you will be passing through all the chakras) until you reach the bottom of the spine. As you are exhaling and lowering your attention down the spine, your eyes can also be lowering and closing. If opening and closing the eyes is not comfortable, don't do this part of the practice until you have more experience with it.
- Hold the breath for a second, then start to inhale slowly. As you inhale, bring your attention upward from the base of the spine to the top of the spine (again you will be passing through all the chakras). As you move upward, your eyes can also be opening slowly.
- Repeat this cycle seven times. One cycle is one trip down and up through the spine.

- Make sure to move slowly while expanding your breath in and out in a controlled manner like you did in full breath.
- After each round, you can take a few yogic breaths and return to do the next round, or you can do the seven rounds continuously.
- At the end of the last round, sit quietly and observe the mind.

Mantra Aum or OM (*Japa*)

Aum and OM are the same mantra. *Au* is pronounced as *O*, and *M* is pronounced on its own. This mantra is the most powerful of all mantras. It is the beginning of all other mantras and holds them all within itself. Just like with the full yogic breath, most people have overlooked this mantra, mistakenly thinking it is a very simple or common mantra. But there is nothing simple about it. There are hidden powers within it that you will come to experience over time.

This practice can be done either audibly or silently.

- Sit comfortably and in a grounded position. Spine is straight.
- Inhale and exhale a few rounds of yogic breath. On the next exhale, with open mouth start to chant *Ooooooooooo*, and three-quarters of the way through the

breath close the lips and continue making the sound *mmmmmmmmm*.

- Then inhale again and repeat the process for five to seven rounds.
- If you are doing the practice silently, you can recite the mantra OM when inhaling and exhaling if you feel comfortable.
- If doing the practice out loud, only repeat the mantra while exhaling.
- When you are finished, sit quietly and observe the mind.

Heart Chakra Meditation (*Anahata Dharana*)
The heart is the seat or home of the divine or higher Self. It is a place we should spend time in, reflect on, and put our mind's focus on as much as possible. Here we find all the answers to our deepest questions and the guidance we are looking for. In this practice, you will focus while using the mantra YAM to help penetrate the heart at the Atmic, or soul, level.

- Sit in a comfortable, stable posture where you don't have to move for a while.
- Close your eyes. Bring the index finger and thumb together and turn your palms upward, placing them on the knees. This mudra invokes consciousness when the

palms face upward; when facing downward they invoke knowledge.

- Take a full yogic breath. Bring your awareness to the heart area. Keep breathing.
- Start to silently repeat the mantra YAM. Chant it as *Yaaaaaaa-mmmmm*, making the *A* and *M* longer. (The *A* is pronounced softly, as though you were saying *YUM*.)Keep breathing and slowly repeat.
- All your focus should be on the heart area in the center of the chest. This is also the location of the anahata chakra.
- Keep breathing slowly, repeating YAM and focusing.
- Do this for five to seven minutes. Don't worry about timing it. You will feel when to stop intuitively.
- After the practice, just sit for a moment.
- Start to listen to the heart.
- Start to feel the heart.
- Notice what your message is from the heart so you act on it today.
- Allow your intuition to guide you. Be open to it by surrendering your mind to it.
- When finishing, bring your awareness or focus from the heart and draw the energy all the way up to look between your eyebrows at the third eye, or ajna chakra, and take a long yogic breath. Close the eyes and observe how you are feeling and how the mind is. After

a few breaths, bring your hands to prayer position in
front of the heart. You are bowing your head to the
teacher inside and being grateful for all the guidance it
is giving you.
+ Remember: if not at this time, many messages and
guidance will be coming to you during the day through
your intuition if you stay tuned in to this frequency you
have created.

This morning practice is just the beginning of the practice
you will now take into the rest of your day. You have created
grounding and supportive energy, which will serve you in every
decision, conversation, and interaction you will encounter. Once
you get used to doing these practices before anything else, it
will soon become a good habit creating more great and healthy
habits.

Make a note and be aware of what kind of energy you feel:

+ Before your practice
+ After your practice
+ During the day
+ At the end of the day

You should also use one or two of these practices at night to
help calm down the mind before sleep.

Used daily, these practices will help you to open up and take you further inward. You won't need any other practices unless you are going to devote more time to do additional practices. If you take more time, you can extend the length of each practice to make them longer, and then over time you can add practices from this book, the twenty-one-day plan, and YCMembership.com.

Self-Study: The Key to Who You Are

I remember the very first book I ever read on spirituality, which was called something like *Knowing Yourself*. This was around 1986, and it was a book I kept rereading over and over again. The cover had a photo of a clear blue sky and a single beautiful cloud in the middle of it. I have never seen that book again. It was a book that was channeled by an entity through someone.

Thinking about it now, I realize that single cloud represented me (or you), and the clear blue sky represented life. We are like a cloud in the sky among many other clouds, but at times we find ourselves alone in the vastness of life. However, we are never actually alone, because we are supported by the sky, which is always holding us within it.

I must have read that book twenty times; it resonated and spoke to me so much. It was asking me not to question but to accept and observe. Not to try to fix or solve issues but to see there were no issues. Not to look for answers but to listen more carefully.

To never separate but to be one. To let things be and see the higher truth within and to know myself.

As I kept reading it, every word just made me feel limitless and free. At some point the words seemed to actually come from within me and not the book, as if they were appearing on the page as I was thinking exactly the same thing.

There are no coincidences in life. Everything and every action has a meaning and perfect place through a greater purpose than what the mind understands. This book came to speak the exact words my mind needed to read and listen to. "When the student is ready, the teacher will appear," goes the ancient saying. But this teacher is not always in the form of a person, but perhaps a book, a child, a beggar, the wind, the sun, or just the breath. In other words, the teacher is everywhere and in everyone. It's all in how you view the teachings.

Discovering Your Higher Self

The higher Self or divine nature is within us all. Did you think for a moment self-study was about you? Of course you did. It's only normal, because we live in a society where we are taught to worship the body and revere the mind. This places our attention on being motivated by self-satisfaction and gives us a sense of self-importance.

All this attention from others starting at a young age gives us a sense of our small self. It emphasizes our material body and mind and inadvertently contributes to self-awareness, drawing our attention outward. Very young children don't have limitations or prejudices, as they have no expectations or judgments. They just observe and take in their surroundings and mainly copy their parents' behaviors. Because we still don't speak at this age, we take in tones and gestures even when we don't know what is being said. All these interactions keep getting absorbed and dig us deeper into the material outer world as we slowly forget the godliness that we came from when we were born. This is how we move from knowing the Self to being selfish.

As we grow up and become more distracted by the outer world, our connection with the inner Self starts to fade, and our awareness of the small self or mind takes hold. This small self, and especially the ego aspect, has a big influence over the mind. It reflects onto the mind many misconceptions, which the intellect thinks are true. This gives us a very one-sided emotional and intellectual experience that is mostly selfish and self-centered. This is because the mind is only interested in gaining importance, power, and control in its current way of thinking. The control the ego is seeking is of other beings and the outer material nature.

Looking at our world today, we can see the evidence of this in our own personal lives as well as around the globe. From the way we communicate to the way we govern, the ego is at play in all of us in some small or very big way. This is evident in how corporations make decisions supposedly for the good of the people, but in fact the decisions are based on what is better for them. On a personal level, it isn't as evident to us how our mind is doing the same. But on a smaller scale, especially in situations when we speak to others or through the thoughts we are having, we tend to have self-interest at heart.

Think about the many circumstances when you speak to someone and how you expect them to understand and respect you, or other times when you feel you need validation. What about times when you judge a situation or someone, when you criticize or compliment someone? If you go through all these scenarios and reflect on all that you think about in, say, just a six-hour period, you will definitely find that nearly all your thoughts in some way circle back to you. It may seem that we are discussing someone else, but underneath the many conversations and opinions we will find that our intentions are very self-centered. This is how the ego is free and loose in the playground of our minds, just running about unaccompanied, screaming and shouting for attention.

We start to control the breathing in our pranayama practices so that we can move beyond the limited functions of the body. Similarly, we can push past the old, limited impressions of the mind by starting to devote our focus back to the light of our higher Self. This will cast such brightness over the ego that it will fade from its darkness and merge into the light.

The higher Self is also called the witness, soul, intuition, super-consciousness, cosmic consciousness, divine, or God. The reason we want to study this energy or power is because it holds the key to our existence, so we need to access, use, and eventually merge with it. It is the energy of the universe within us. It is beyond all and it is all. It is omnipotent, omnipresent, and omniscient. It is beyond all thought and beyond the normal comprehension of the mind or senses. It is who we truly are when the ego is quiet.

The majority of humans are living the "fake self." The imposter. The pretender. The human race has been kidnapped by the mind and is living a kind of illusion while acting like we are all immortal. We are living on the surface of life in the most materialistic ways possible by indulging the senses to their maximum while speaking of searching for the deeper meaning of things like happiness, God, and love.

When I was nineteen and working in the fashion world, I was a perfect example of someone living on the surface but speaking about spiritual teachings. My focus was on having a good time, making money, and maximizing my exposure to fame, but I was also reading many spiritual books and understood many of the philosophies and teachings. I was not a daily practitioner yet, but rather an amateur spiritualist who loved to have spiritual discussions.

I would say spirituality was my favorite topic of conversation. I remember bringing it up in pretty much all the conversations I had, whether I was talking about fashion, beauty, or anything else. It just spoke to me so deeply. But while I was speaking about the Self, I also needed to know more about myself. I remember when I started my first teacher training in New York City we had to study *The Yoga Sutras* of Patanjali (my book *The One Plan* is a practical guide to these teachings), and in the *Yoga Sutras* one of the teachings is about self-study.

As I read more about it, I understood that I also needed to know more about myself while on the path to uniting with the higher Self. So I thought it would be a good idea to speak to my parents about my childhood and what I was like. I thought this would give me an insight to what kind of behavior and background made up my character and personality, and why my mind thinks the way it does.

First, my father and mother are not particularly interested in chatting about spirituality, although they had to endure many of my conversations over the years. They endured with dignity and patience, as most parents might have just said, "We love you, but please shut up or change the subject."

I asked them many questions about the situations we had gone through together and my reactions to them. As we lived in Iran and had some beautiful times and some very difficult times together, how we all reacted to these various situations was of great interest to me. Apparently, I have always been a little mischievous but always polite and calm. And I loved to play a lot, playing with the neighborhood kids, and I was fearless running through local grape farms full of snakes.

I was raised to not have fear of any race, gender, or religion. Although people looked as if they were of different colors, they were actually all the same color with different shades. I saw all people at the same economic level. Politics, religion, and money were never discussed at home, as they were seen as the root of all conflict.

So when I look back at the way I was brought up and how that shaped my nature from birth to adulthood, I see many insights into why I think about, view, and react to the world as I do. Next I looked over all the aspects of myself that I found useful and positive and decided to keep those. Then I focused on the aspects, habits, and thoughts that I had no more use for and started to work on changing those through the yogic practices that I was learning. This is how you put these practices into action and begin to discover your higher Self.

All the practices we do on this path are to move through levels. Like an athlete who is training to run his best race and conquer every step, we are continuously training and moving through different states of awareness, reaching toward our inner and higher Self. It is an invisible path we are traveling on, but the journey is clear. Once you start your journey, all you need is dedication to the practices and a deep desire to know your maker. The rest you can leave up to the divine to guide and accompany you on your journey.

The great thing about the yogic path is that wherever you are in your life, you can join in. No one is really at the beginning, because as you have been living your life you have also applied certain yogic values or principles without knowing it. You may find that moving from a physical level to a more subtle form takes time for you. But if you go at a sustainable pace so that you never stop practicing, then you will be living as a yogi. You will be jogging a marathon and not sprinting the hundred meters.

The Path of Self-Surrender

Self-surrender is a whole yogic path on its own. It brings us patience and relief from having to be "someone." It takes us to the understanding that we are someone already and we just need to focus on who we are by surrendering the small self to the higher Self. In the same way a devotee follows and surrenders to the guru or master, here we surrender our ego mind to the guru within. It is the acknowledgment that something greater than our body or mind exists. It is the bowing down to something higher in a universe unseen but discoverable by way of faith and sincere devotion. Without this surrender and humbleness we can never arrive at our goal of being free from all the conflicts of the mind.

For us to understand greater truths and arrive at the answers to the higher questions in life, we have to surrender ourselves and be like children who are listening to and following every vibration that the inner voice is guiding them toward. You will not hear this guidance until you start to trust that quieter voice beneath the louder one. You describe it as having a hunch or gut feeling, and this of course is what we call our intuition. Intuition is also the Self. As we surrender the small self to the big Self through the use of our spiritual practices, we allow the subtle sound to be more audible. Trusting our intuition takes practice. Through sense control and concentration practices, observation of ourselves, and changes to our habits, together with slowing down and contemplating more—we start trusting and following our intuition with confidence. We start to distinguish between one voice and the other.

Of course this becomes easier as we practice on a daily basis. And at times we will feel like we are sailing calm and tranquil waters and the ego has gone away for good, which is a big mistake. This little pest never actually leaves our mind but just keeps hiding and switching disguises. This is why we must practice daily, to help tame the ever-changing mind.

How do you know whether you are following the ego mind or your intuition? This is very easy to distinguish. The ego is always loud and creates confusion in the mind. It wants one thing, then at the same time it wants exactly the opposite. It loves and it hates. It cries and then it is happy. It is insecure, then it is arrogant. It is dualistic and excessive in everything. You have all experienced this when trying to make decisions and your mind is dragging you through all the options to choose something, be it a new job, what to eat for lunch, or when to leave for a trip. With the ego there is always self-interest or self-doubt in everything we choose.

Our intuition is exactly the opposite. It never changes direction and it is always consistent. It doesn't go from one extreme to the other. It is content and detached at all times. It is the voice that guides with gentle and loving kindness. It is that voice that you always come back to even if you never followed its direction in the first place. It is always the first voice we hear before the mind comes in and starts chatting. It is not always the voice of reason or what the mind wants to hear, but the guide to what is correct for us even when there is an easier way out.

I was Skyping with one of my clients, asking how she was doing. She told me she was frustrated because they sent her robot to the wrong address. My client is a robotics scientist, so I knew what she was talking about; otherwise I might have thought she had been watching too many *Star Wars* movies. I ask her to elaborate a little.

She told me she had been rushing to get her invention into a competition, and the delivery company sent it to a farm and missed the delivery address by a few hundred miles. I started to laugh a little at the notion that a farmer has a robot, probably baffled about what to do with it.

Now my work here was to have my client seek the truth and understand the higher meaning of her experience, so she could know how to move on. I asked her to give me further details, describing the whole experience up to her mailing the package. It turned out she had been very anxious and rushing to finish the robot but knew it was not really ready yet for the competition. "I knew I shouldn't have sent it. Something was telling me to not send it because it wouldn't work properly."

I asked her what her intention was by entering the robot into the competition. "I just wanted to see how it would do."

This is a clear example of doing something when the intention you have is not clear or strong enough to reach your intended goal, and the main issue is that intuition is speaking loudly, trying to keep the mind from doing something it will regret. My client already knew (intuition) her product wasn't ready, but she decided (the mind) to send it anyway. We (the mind) know that the Self (intuition) has all the answers, but we just like rebelling because it makes us feel like an individual and in control.

In this case, the higher Self intervened (karma) and diverted the robot to a farm, so it didn't reach the competition. Karma means action, and every action has a reaction. This reaction is a result of the action, so it is the karma attached to the action. That way karma is never ending. If the robot did reach the competition, the criticism and judgment it might have received for not working correctly could have had a very negative effect on my client's confidence and emotions, discouraging her from trying again.

The Self knows the mind's limitations and weaknesses and is always trying to protect it, which is why we have to practice self-surrender to our higher consciousness and intuition. Learning to listen and trust what is being communicated from within is a necessary guide for each step we take in life, and my client learned a valuable lesson from having her robot "accidentally" lost, which turned out to be a real blessing in the end.

Self-Observation

Most of our self-observation is about our likes and dislikes. We describe ourselves as different types of people with different preferences. We speak about who we are and what we are not. We like to compare and identify with others we admire. We talk about others and describe their attributes or flaws, their character or personality. All of these types of observations and opinions are information that describes people on the surface level: what colors they prefer, if they are funny or serious, what sexual preference they have, or if they are a vegan or eat meat.

But none of this surface information tells us about the true Self. This surface information is like thick dust that has collected on a tabletop, to the point that you can't see if the tabletop is made of wood, glass, or something else. We have collected so much mental dust that when we meet people, we don't see their true nature as a reflection of the nature within ourselves. We have gotten so used to commenting on how a person looks physically that we totally miss anything deeper about them. Even when we describe someone as spiritual, we are really only describing a trait and not the actual spirit connection one can feel with them, otherwise we wouldn't be comparing them to ourselves or others—that is, until the moment you have a heart connection with someone and feel you have known them for many lifetimes, when actually you have only just met them in this lifetime. These are the moments when we connect soul to soul, moving beyond the mind.

Life is pretty simple for infants. They observe everything and everyone. As children, we didn't have opinions or conflicts with things or people. For instance, as children we see different skin colors as a variation and not as a difference. We feel sexuality but not as a particular category or type. In all we do and hear we have a soul desire to fit in with others and not to be separate from anyone.

But as we become young adults things begin to change. With adults around we start to mirror their beliefs, prejudices, and fears. As we grow older, the mind begins to project these traits outward in our behavior, using a similar language and tone. We start to identify with the differences between us and not so much with the commonalities we share. We become distracted by the exterior of a person and forget about our initial soul-to-soul connection.

From here we begin to learn about fear and separateness in body and mind. And I use the word *learn* because being separate is a state of fear that doesn't come naturally; we have to learn it. Of course inside we still know we are not separate, but because our ego grows in power it casts a greater shadow on our mind. From here we start to choose sides and build fences, putting up doors and walls in our mind, which is the beginning of compartmentalizing other beings into categories and mental boxes.

Our journey of self-observation starts by going through the layers of physical, mental, and spiritual self. We first start to observe our body and evaluate how healthy it is. How is our digestion, elimination, and nervous system? Do we have aches and pains? What are our capabilities? How strong or weak is our willpower? We must take all aspects of our body into account so we can understand our endurance and capacity—how all of our systems work and how clear all the channels in our body are, what elements are more balanced or imbalanced.

We go through this process to be able to feel every aspect of our physical being and to gain mastery over it. This is self-discipline in the physical realm. If we don't have control over the body, then it will take away the attention of the mind and distract us when it is not well. Take, for example, when you have aches and pains. Can you really focus on anything else when your migraine is in full effect? This is why observing the body and keeping it at optimal health is very important.

On the mental level, we start to observe our true nature and how our mind works. We notice if our mind is calm, very active, or very passive. What are the most important things on our mind that we think about continuously? What are our beliefs and what motivates us? What are our preferences and how far are we willing to go to get what we want? How dedicated are we to our cause or direction in life? Do we have peace or are we always agitated?

These observations begin to reveal everything about the way our mind works, its attachments, and its thought patterns. We become an observer of every movement and thought we have. The way we think will be a huge determining factor in the way our life turns out. This is why it is so important to know yourself very well on the mental level.

Over time, as we observe everything there is to see or feel with our physical, mental, and emotional self through our body and mind, we start to become aware of our inner energy through the practice of contemplation. Asking questions and contemplating becomes our way of self-inquiry: we question our existence on earth and in the universe; what it means to be a human among other living beings; what it means to die and leave the body. We want to understand why we are here and why the spirit has chosen to go through this human birth in this particular form, to understand how Mother Nature works and how we are just like her, made from exactly the same vibration and energy.

As we go through this process of contemplation, we start to get a better sense of our small surface self and the meaning of our existence beyond just the material form. As we start to expand the mind to the point it can't go further, that's when we realize we need the assistance of something higher to understand deeper knowledge. This is when we reach toward our higher Self through yogic practices.

Try this practice right now to better understand what I am speaking about, because I know spiritual talk can get very abstract and it takes practice to reveal the meaning behind it. The tools you will use for this practice of self-study are contemplation, observation, and awareness.

Observe the state of your health. Does your body command your attention a lot? Does it get your attention because you want a better body, want to lose weight, or have aches, pains, or an ailment? How much time do you spend thinking about your body?

Now become aware of your mind. What are the top five thoughts on your mind each day: family, children, work, money, politics, power, control, fear, desire, music, spirituality, fashion, beauty, and so on? Whatever is taking up your mind space is determining how your self is turning out. And how you are reacting to all these thoughts is determined by your nature, which we discussed in the last chapter on practice.

Your nature is the one you were born with, so when it comes

to your reactions they mainly follow your childhood patterns. If, for example, you are thinking about money, and you were raised in a comfortable home with no money worries, then your thoughts might be of abundance, spending freely without fear. But another person who has had a more frugal upbringing might never feel like they have enough (even if they do), so they always worry about money: same financial status and lifestyle, but different mind-sets and nature.

Now you can apply this contemplation practice to every thought in your mind. Observe how the thoughts you are having are influencing your life so you can make changes and shifts. Unless you understand yourself (the mind, thoughts, memories, and reactions), you will not be able to move forward to higher thinking. This is the yogic process a yogi is taking every moment as we are bombarded with outer stimulations and old sense memory. It truly is a battlefield in our minds where we don't know when the enemy will attack but we know they will.

Study of Spiritual Material

Another way of helping ourselves along the path of self-discovery is to read, study, and contemplate spiritual content through books, seminars, courses, and workshops. Engaging our senses, mind, and intellect with written and verbal practices helps us connect with different messages and teachings that we learn to adapt to. As we hear and read ancient teachings, our minds begin to recollect from within what the truth of existence is. All the surface conversations and everyday life chatter begin to fade, replaced with an understanding of deeper awareness. The small talk in our subconscious gets replaced with images of divine lessons and truths of our soul's journey and path up to this point.

As we keep reading, studying, and practicing on a daily basis, we are reminded of the higher power and divine consciousness that lies within and that our world outside is only one level of existence and only real to the mind as long as we are in the body. When our soul or spirit transcends the body, then the material level becomes an illusion that once was but is no more. The more authentic the teachings that we follow, the better we will be guided and catapulted into higher thinking and higher living. These teachings shouldn't take us deeper into the mind with intellectual talk but should help release our mind through spiritual practices.

Almost every aspect of our modern-day lifestyle takes our attention outside of ourselves, so daily reading as part of a spiritual practice brings our attention back inward. Because at our subtlest level we are spirit energy, and because the spirit is the all seer and knower of the entire universe, it already has every bit of information, knowledge, and wisdom that exists.

The spiritual reading we do should be 10 percent inspirational, 20 percent instructional, and 70 percent practical. This way we will be under no illusion that discovering the "secret" is the answer to all our issues or dreams. We understand that discovering the secret door is just the beginning of the journey, as the next steps are how to open the door by having the right code, and then taking the path waiting on the other side. In the same way, when we learn how to swim or train for a new job, we first get excited, then we get instructions, and then we spend most of the time actually performing the action to master the skill. Remember never to get lost in just reading or talking spirituality. Reading and discussing are only a support to practice and never take the place of practice, otherwise all you will have is theory without the experience.

Chapter Summary

- Higher Self and the self are two different aspects of what we call "us."
- Intuition doesn't doubt or change its message. The mind does.
- Look into your childhood conditioning so you know what thought patterns are holding you back and which ones serve you best.

• Place less attention on the physical body and focus on
  the mind and intuition.

Daily Life Practice

1. To reach and live a higher state of consciousness, speak
   less, read more, and above all practice everything you
   read, because it is the practice and not the speaking or
   reading that is going to make your life spiritual.
2. When you wake up in the morning, recall or even keep
   a journal of your dreams. As part of knowing yourself
   better, you also need to know what the mind is thinking during sleep time. Many of our fears and conflicts
   come out and can be resolved during this time at
   night.
3. Sit right now for just five minutes and reflect on the
   thoughts you are having and what the content of this
   chapter has stirred up for you. When reading about self-
   study the mind really starts to ponder itself, which is an
   interesting time to observe what sits well with you and
   what your mind is uncomfortable with. This is getting
   to know yourself inside out.
4. Every day ask yourself: "Who am I?" Just sit for a quiet
   moment and reflect. Doing this over time will take you

deeper into contemplation of your higher Self. But you have to ask with love and compassion, as this is the language the heart responds to.

5. When you meet people, even if you know them already, look beyond their body and see what their heart is saying to you. Every encounter is a chance to have a soul-to-soul connection and move beyond the surface chatter.

Intention: The Key to Manifest

Most people think they know what their intentions are. But we don't most of the time. I know I didn't when I first set out on the yogic path. I just knew it was a path that had the same values and goals I was interested in—liberation on a spiritual level. But this was only a mental knowing at this point. For most of my life, I didn't know my intentions. I didn't really know what it meant, and so throughout my life I did things because I wanted to but not really understanding why.

When I was a model, I wanted to have a good time and travel the world. But can I say I really consciously intended to do that? I definitely put my energy into having a good time and traveling, but most of it was unconscious. I don't really remember living in a conscious and intentional way until I started to have a daily yogic practice.

This was when I started to ask myself the questions "Why am I doing this?" and "What are my intentions for it?" From the beginning of my ayurveda and yoga training, I wanted to be an ambassador for this way of living. I get so much peace and direction from this lifestyle that I wanted everyone to feel what I am feeling. But I have also gotten distracted many times along my path.

While I started with that higher intention as an overall direction, I have also been affected by my circumstances, environment, and life in general, so at times my attention went toward money or selfish thoughts. I have been distracted by others and picked projects that I had no intention of finishing. Experience is a great tool to have because we can reflect on it and make better decisions as we go forward.

So from my experience, I now make decisions based on an intention that whatever I do in work, family, or community needs to be of benefit for all. I fall short at times and things are not perfect as I would like them to be, but I now have a clear intention and direction for what I do. My intentions are influenced by my responsibility to the world as a community and environment, to others, and to myself. This means my intentions and duty need to be the same.

We all have many good or personal intentions, but are we taking the actions that correspond to living out those intentions? We still need to take an action in order for our intentions to have meaning and come into being. Just having intentions on their own doesn't give them any power to manifest. This is why good intentions are just 10 percent of the journey or the inspirational factor.

The other 90 percent is all the work you have to put in to your intentions for them to have any success.

The Key That Opens All Doors

The word *sankalpa* has different definitions, but they are all descriptions of the same process: know your intentions, take action, and watch them manifest. It sounds simple, and it is. You are already practicing this formula in everyday life: when you say to yourself, "I am going to yoga class tomorrow at 7:00 A.M.," and you follow through and do it. Or when you crave pancakes and promise to make them for breakfast the next day and you do—this is living out your intentions. This is sankalpa on a basic, short-term level.

You might have practiced sankalpa as a long-term goal when you promised yourself to stay in college and graduate no matter how hard things became. Or said to yourself that you would travel to Africa as soon as you had the money and did so after many years. Sankalpa is an intention that you really intend to carry out and see through. It's not a flippant remark, gesture, or fancy idea that comes and goes. It's a solid inner intention that is ingrained in us, and no matter what our distractions are we never waver or become sidetracked from it, even if it takes many years to achieve.

Most things in life that we say we are going to do never actually happen. This is because we are not following through with the process of bringing them to fruition. Ideas without the correct intentions are powerless. It's not enough for us to wish or sit and wait for things to come without putting the power of intention and action behind them. The energy of just talking about something is dormant and average; it isn't supercharged with power and direction. It lacks the drive needed to bring something into an energetic form.

Everything in the universe is energy in the form of sound and light, and energy vibrates at different levels. Vibrations have individual movements that create particular outcomes. When we have a certain conviction and drive, it is energy in motion. It shows us how the intention first starts in the mind, thoughts, and psyche, where it builds and gains momentum. From here it grows in strength through creative action, where eventually the intention starts to manifest on the material plane. Without first being a seed thought in our mind, an intention lacks strength to become reality. Like a seed that first needs planting, watering, and eventually nurturing to become the plant it will grow into, our intentions need to first become thoughts, watered with daily contemplation and eventually nurtured with passion and willpower so they can thrive into being.

There are two places sankalpa is being directed from:

1. Intentions coming from the purest level, where our focus and determination is driven by our heart's desire. It is a soul desire that puts into motion greatness on a spiritual level that benefits all beings and is inclusive. It is selfless and uninterested in the outcome or fruits of labor for personal gain. There is no separateness or individuality in it. It is a vibration that unites, knowing that everything belongs to all, not just one. On this higher level, the vibration created by our intentions attracts other souls with the same vibratory intentions. This creates a circuit of energy, which is shared, endless, and part of the universal consciousness.

2. Intentions directed from our mind's desire. Here we create an individual and separate energy that is recognized in the material world as personal achievement and not as a universal one. This energy carries with it the vibration of individual ego "greatness." This then creates imbalance in us and for others; it complicates life and creates things like disease and pollution, as we are experiencing with many of humanity's inventions so far. Sankalpa on this lower level may bring praise and awards, which lead to material gain, but it does not bring higher loving energy for all to share. Like the

hundred-meter race that is over in a blink of an eye, so glory on this path does not last long.

Setting a path of spiritual sankalpa with balance is to be inclusive of all beings and to take the earth into our highest consideration. We have spiritual foresight when we have an idea and start an intention to see if it is coming from a heart desire or a mind desire; to see what kind of impact our intentions will have on Mother Nature, which feeds and sustains us.

As we walk the yogi path, we learn to discern and recognize if our intentions will harm others or be of service to them. Is our intention to maximize our personal profits or to be of service? If our ideas meet these higher Self standards, then we can continue to make them happen, knowing we have the full support of the divine creator from within—and, more important, that we are living out the soul's purpose and avoiding more lifetimes of suffering. It is not to say that the Self will not also help bring our ego desires into being too, but when we focus our intention with the aim to serve others there is balance among what we want, what we give, and what we receive in return.

Most of our world up to now, especially the last few thousand years, has been fashioned from our inner ego desires. This is why we compete, challenge, destroy, fight, and build things that in the short term seem a good creative idea but in the long run bring more suffering to everyone because they were never created from the balanced higher energy. It's not that the higher path of sankalpa is better than the lower path of mind desires, but it will have different outcomes and effects on our life, being, and karma.

For instance, the inventors of the cell phone or a brand of soda might have thought their ideas would change the world in a positive way by connecting the world and bringing some joy to people's palates. Or they might have just wanted to make a successful brand and express their creative power. Whatever their intention was, only they really know, but we can see the effects of what these products have had on people's health and well-being. So even if an intention was initially "good," the outcome can be negative, because the intention is coming from our mind or ego and not our heart.

Mind Versus Divinely Driven Intention

If our intention is to benefit every being and at the same time make use of but not abuse Mother Nature, then our ideas and intentions will have the highest desired effect and benefit for all beings. Our idea will reflect our intention when brought into action. As we live in a world of commerce, business, and capitalism, it is one of our biggest challenges to be able to make a living and adhere to this principle and higher cause. Everywhere we look we can see the evidence and effects of the ego-invention intentions being fulfilled. And our society is perpetuating and driving these ideas and products forward by consuming them without much awareness. But when it comes to spiritual and healthy intentions and inventions, we still lack diversity because we are limited by the economic factors that say we must make large profits to deem something worthy or to even make it sustainable to stay in business. These are the modern-day challenges we face together.

Can we stop an intention once we have taken the action to bring it into reality? Bringing sankalpa into every aspect of our life, we can see that every action we take has some sort of personal intention behind it. Once we have taken the action to put our intention into motion, it is too late to change some of the outcome because part of the energy is already taking shape. It's like sending a current of electricity down a cable. Even if we decide to turn it off, we have still directed some amount of current down the cable and we can't stop it. We can always change our mind or thoughts and change our intention, but depending on how long we have been setting an intention, that amount of energy will be behind it.

And the effects of our intentions also live on for much longer than maybe we had intended. We may have also already changed our mind, but the effects of our intentions live on, as they are energy. It's like saying something and using certain words. They have an effect on others for much longer than the time it took to say them. We might have changed our point of view, but the effects of the original words or actions still live on. This is why people are endlessly apologizing for things they have said or done. But if the intention behind apologizing is to be sincere, then the apology means something and has an intended healing affect. And if we are just apologizing with the intention of being polite or showing good face, then it is meaningless and has a superficial effect.

Most people don't understand why a certain part of their life advances relatively well while another part is mostly unpredictable or unstable. People usually just do things and then think about them later, or don't think about them at all. For example, when you turn on the TV, do you think about why you want to watch TV, beyond just thinking of a show you want to see? Do you turn on the TV and think, "Why am I watching TV?" Usually you just turn it on without considering your intention, although there is an intention behind the action. The hidden reason might be because you are bored, alone, want to be entertained, need some noise on, have an attachment to a show or celebrity, or a host of other reasons you are not aware of.

So most of the time we are without direction and an understanding of why we take the actions we do. This is especially true of today's modern-day fast world, where people feel they are just playing catch-up with all the work, family, and other things they have to do. Who really has time to stop to think about why they do something?

One of the main reasons to stop and contemplate our reason for doing something is that it usually saves a lot of time and energy much later when the outcome of the action has taken place. If, for example, you don't first understand why you are entering a relationship, marriage, or partnership, somewhere down the line when things are not going as smoothly as they used to, you may start to have major issues and perhaps even a breakup simply because you never knew why you were in the partnership in the first place.

So maybe because you didn't set an intention, didn't do a little contemplation, and didn't understand the reason behind your decision to enter a partnership, you have to spend the next few years suffering the aftereffects of it all. This is where sankalpa saves us a lot of time and unnecessary suffering, taking us directly to where we need to be without any distractions. A few days of thinking and setting intentions can save many years of effort trying to undo a big mess. It's one of the best investments of time, with a great return in peacefulness and clarity.

Right now, for instance, you could examine the reason you chose the job you are doing. Do you have great interest in your work? Is it a part of your conscious lifestyle? Does it add to humanity and the greater good of all? Is it simply financial? Do you have any idea why you do this job?

Spend a few minutes being honest about why you do your job. Ask yourself if it is a job or your life's work. This way you will know your intention for why you do your job and why you behave the way you do at work. Our intentions for why we do something affect our attitude and behavior toward it.

*

Our ideas and intentions say a lot about what's going on in our mind and thoughts. They are the reflections of our mind in the same way our lifestyle and habits reflect the way we choose to live. How we are living, the lifestyle we follow, and the choices we make are directly related to our innermost feelings and wants. This isn't always evident to us because when we think about what we want, our answer usually doesn't match our current situation. "I want a more successful career, I want to make more money, I want children, I want to be understood, I want to be loved."

But are we taking the actions for these things to happen? And are these things we really want? More often than not, our deepest desires are not the same as what we speak about on the surface. We may think and talk about having a big career, but actually deep down we are avoiding it because we don't want to work too hard or we don't do well under pressure. How many times have we said one thing and turned around and done the opposite? And then later complained about it?

There are no coincidences as to why this happens. It is because we are not clear about what we really want and what we are willing to do to get it.

Knowing Your Intentions—Knowing Yourself

In the last chapter we discussed self-study and learning the difference between our small self and higher Self. To know ourselves and all our tendencies, habits, and attitudes toward life teaches us a great deal about the intentions we have and will be drawn toward. Our nature influences our intentions, and our intentions reflect our nature. When someone comments that you did something out of character, it is because they don't know your true inner intentions in that moment. They are only going by what they know about you on the surface, but not what intentions you have or have had for many years. Isn't this true when you hear someone comment that they would never have guessed so-and-so could ever do such a thing? Or that someone never keeps their promise?

Each one of us comes into the world with a particular individual nature that becomes our own character DNA. Our body and mind pretty much function just like everyone else's, but our personal nature is different. As our nature interacts with people and the environment, it gathers and stores different stories, feelings, memories, and information that we develop into our own specific habits based on how our "filter" works. This is how from a young age we already set many of our sankalpas and our deepest desires to reach certain goals. Depending on how extreme life has been and how our character has digested it all, we will have developed a particular character. The more extreme events and life experiences we have been through, the deeper and more concrete many of our intentions become.

For example, if we came from a family that experienced our parents fighting and splitting up, then one of our parents going through a lot of emotional or financial hardship, we may have at that time vowed to be very different from our parents. We might decide to be disciplined, never to argue with our future partner, and to work hard never to have financial issues or depend on another person. This is a story many will relate to. But few may have actually carried this through unless it really scared their mind to an extreme point that it did not stop being a priority and a driving force throughout their adulthood. This is an example of a deep-seated intention set many years before that is fueled by our personal experience and driven by our individual nature.

In the same scenario, another person might think they are setting the same resolve to become very disciplined and to never abandon a relationship, but their character lacks the determination or real interest. So the intention this person sets loses direction and energy; it never comes to fruition simply because they didn't truly set a strong and concrete intent in the first place. This person would probably be less hurt and emotional about the whole ordeal, being more forgiving and understanding. This attitude dissipates a lot of a person's resentment or frustrations, and in the process any strong intention to retaliate or to prove something to themselves or others gradually fades away.

Setting New Intentions and Changing Old Ones

There are old, deep-rooted intentions we set many years ago that are known or unknown to us, but we can also set new intentions for ourselves based on what we want in life. To set new and fresh intentions or to ignite an old, stale intention, there are several things to consider:

1. Is your intention being guided from the mind or the intuitive Self?
2. Do you have a deep belief in your intention?
3. Is the intention in line with your true nature and character?
4. Are you willing to stick with it even if it takes many years to achieve?

First, know where your intentions are coming from. If they are from the ego, then be okay with it unless you are trying to reach higher goals. Some people who read spiritual material or follow some of the yogic teachings work against themselves because they feel guilty if they prosper from wealth gained from a selfish, mind-driven level. Don't be. Guilt is a waste of precious life, and if your nature is more ego driven, don't feel bad about it. Yes, you should always be trying to do better, but each person's definition of better varies according to what they know and understand.

One morning I was speaking about this to a friend. She was telling me how bad she felt about selling meat in her business as she was turning to vegetarianism. Her business sold meat products, but she didn't believe in eating meat. This is a dualistic situation where a person is not clear or committed to their new intention but is still holding on to their older and deeper one. I explained to her that for her to be able to move forward without any guilt or negative energy, she should either stick to her present business model until she was ready for a shift or commit to the change straightaway if she felt this was a lifestyle commitment she was making for life. I told her to contemplate it for a while so the real truth for her could come to the surface naturally.

Second, do you have a deep inner intention for what you want to embark on, or is it just a surface idea? Ideas are many, but intentions should be few and very selective, especially long-term sankalpa. If we are selective with our long-term intentions we are less likely to get confused or frustrated that they are not happening quickly enough. This is because we will not have set too many unrealistic goals. Many short-term commitments can be met quicker, as they don't need as much thought and planning. But the long-term and more significant goals that are fewer but require much more time and effort over many years need to be cultivated with real, true commitment.

Third, is your intention in line with your true inner character and nature? As observed before, we have a certain character and nature that is very individual to us and no one else. Part of this has to do with the karma we have created in this and our past lives. Karma plays a major role in our life, as every action or thought we have ever had has created and continues to create reactions—over and over. These actions and reactions are our personal karma. This karma has helped shape the person we are today and the life we are living.

It is our job to contemplate and start to put aside anything we have intended to do that does not go with our personality or character. For example, you are a very creative person who is free spirited, but because you think you need to make quick money you decide to take a job in an office. You know deep down this is not going to be a place you will thrive. This would be an intention to put aside and forget about so you don't distract yourself anymore. It would be productive to move away from all things that you have been thinking about that are not in line with your belief, path, and character and start to focus on the one or two things that are very much in line with your personality. Ideas need energy behind them so they can become alive and living.

Lastly, are you willing to stick with things for the long term? Once you identify the one or two projects that are very much about you and your personality, it is time to see if they are realistic and attainable. Maybe you have thought about opening a restaurant because you love food, you like the social aspect, and you want to write cookbooks. But do you know how much work goes into operating a successful restaurant and how many hours you have to dedicate to it? If you don't, then you would need to speak to someone who does.

You would need to sit and observe or even work in a restaurant for a few weeks to understand the scope of what it takes: the hours, the interaction, the financials, etc. Once you have this information you will have to contemplate if your character would be able to cope with the load and thrive in a restaurant environment. It's one thing to want to own a restaurant and another to run it daily. But again, for any endeavor you want to pursue, you will have to look into this very important detail: is it in my nature to stick with this activity, work, or project that I am about to begin?

This is how you live the "authentic you."

I know from many of my own endeavors, especially before I embarked on the yogic path, that all the activities that were outside the bounds of my character fell to the side pretty quickly. My energy could not sustain and bring the activity into reality, even though my mind had the right intention in that moment. My overall failure rate has been much greater than my success rate.

The potential for our intention to manifest lies directly in our clear focus on our goal and why we want to make a particular commitment to a path or cause. When we value our time we will never waste it on anything that does not fall in line with our lifestyle, character, or true beliefs.

Every Action Has Intention

Even if you don't know it at the time, there is always a reason for everything. Absolutely everything that happens in your life, the world, and the universe has a purpose and reason. It's just that we don't always know the reason, or often don't want to recognize the reason for all the things that happen in the world and the universe, which are much bigger than our personal existence.

But we should be aware of why things happen to us on an individual level. For this to happen and for us to be very aware of why our life is heading in one direction or another, we have to become conscious of our little and bigger intentions on all physical, mental, and spiritual levels.

We have very distinctive intentions set from when we were children that are in our psyche to this very day and we have set some subtle thoughts to read this book and do some other things. On a physical level we set intentions to get in better shape and lose weight. We think about eating less and much better. We vow to do a cleanse and become healthy. These are all thoughts that people have in their regular life. On a mental level, we are constantly making plans to do things (which are like small sankalpas); especially when we are stressed or have anxious thoughts that are full of fear, we are setting some sort of intention for the near future.

Say you are at work and your company has merged with another company and there are going to be layoffs. Even before anyone has been let go, your mind goes into a commentary on how you will be one of the first to go, and for weeks you have these thoughts in your mind. Without even being aware of it, through your fear you are setting yourself up to be fired because your mantra has become "I'm going to get fired."

You see, in repeating the same words or activity, they become a mantra and inadvertently become our intention in motion, knowingly or unknowingly. There are many hidden intentions we perpetuate that we are not aware of, but each one affects our life: every time we say we are going to get back at someone or we are going to do something nice for someone, we are setting intentions in motion.

On a spiritual level we also set intentions, but maybe much less on this level than on the others. The spiritual level isn't always as tangible as the physical body or mental realms. If we are spiritually conscious of the divine within us through our practice, then we understand that everything we do and say brings energy with it. But intuitive intentions are part of a spiritual life, as our ideas, thoughts, and sankalpa are very intentional and not left up to chance. This level is the highest level of intuitive consciousness, as sankalpa is a natural way of living and a part of our lifestyle choices.

Moving Forward from This Moment

Start to make every step of your life a conscious movement of intentions. Today, before you eat, first become aware of your intention. Be aware whether you are going to eat out of real hunger, boredom, pleasure, entertainment, or a desire to socialize. Before you speak, before a word leaves your mouth, understand your intention behind saying something. Be conscious if you are speaking out of truth, fear, ambition, anger, or joy. The next meeting you go to, question your intent. Are you going to get something, to be of service, or to share in a moment?

Apply this way of thinking to everything you do and see the truth behind everything that motivates you. See how surprised you become when you first check your motivation and intent behind your next action. As you apply this to any situation in life—family, friends, work, and all your personal habits—a clear picture will emerge of how you became the person you are today, why you do the things you do, and where you are heading in the next twenty years. As you get into the habit of first checking your motivations and intentions, slowly you will start to head in a direction that is preferable to you and old habits will turn into new and productive ones.

Right now, I know from my own life that I am motivated and have an intention to be productive in everything I do. My interactions all have to be specifically about growing on my path and sharing time with others who want to enter this path or advance further along it. I was not always like this, and for now it is a phase of my path while I am working with people. Maybe when I settle into village life many years from now, my intention will be to do more practice and not have as much interaction. For now this is my reality, which I have created through my intentions.

This is a sure way of paving your old road with new asphalt of conscious intentions, where you know why you are doing something and what your expectations are. You may still not always get what you want, but you will know for sure why you did something without any confusion or regrets. It makes for a much clearer mind and more guiltless existence.

Chapter Summary

- Make use of your experiences before making decisions to do something.

- Are you following a mind intention or an intuitive heart intention?
- There is no easy way, just the right way, which your intentions set out.
- Focus more on your deep intentions and not just the short-term, surface ones.
- Understand what you are motivated by so you can live your intention fully.

Daily Life Practice

Contemplate these questions for ten to fifteen minutes a day and fill in the answers. For you to move forward with clarity of intention, a little time needs to be invested in knowing what sits behind every action you want to take. Come back and read your answers in a month, three months, or one year and see if your answers are still the same or if they have changed.

1. Intentions need energy and action behind them to bring them to fruition. How much are you willing to do to bring your deepest intentions into being? Are you willing to work six, eight, or ten hours a day? Seven days a week if necessary? Are you willing to forgo vacations with your family? Knowing these answers will allow

you to set realistic goals so success is attainable and not an unrealistic, distant dream.

2. Why do you speak and think the way you do? What do you repeat every day, which has become your mantra? "I can," "I will," "when possible," "not now," "sure, soon," or "when I get the time"? Change your mantra to what it needs to be for you to reach your goal.

3. What is the intention of your life? To find happiness, to be successful, to be loved, to be liberated, etc.? This is your big, long-term goal. What are you doing to work toward this goal? What are you doing that is working against it?

4. How has your true nature influenced your intentions and the way you live today, making choices as you do?

5. Do the words you speak match your intentions? If not, change your dialogue to match your intentions, and watch your intentions come to life.

Purpose: The Key to Your Life's Destiny

My ultimate life purpose has been to walk the yogic path. I know this through the intuition that speaks to me, but before I started on this path I had no idea what my purpose was—not my true soul's purpose. I had such an amazing time in the fashion world that I didn't think life could get any better. I knew about the spiritual world, but I had no experience of it, or maybe I never recognized it.

The outer world seemed just fine to me. It was exciting and I didn't need to be purposeful except for the purpose of having a beautiful and fun time. Outer beauty, outer recognition, outer fun, outer love, and outer peace all became what I thought were my purpose. Life seemed to be just perfect the way it was; after all, everyone I met wanted that same kind of exciting life that I was living.

I also see that my whole life has been a preparation to enter this path. If you asked me when I was nineteen what kind of person would likely be a yogi, I first would have asked you to explain what

a yogi is. Then my guess would have been a monk living in seclu-
sion in the Himalayas, or someone who was born into a family of
gurus in an ashram. But this all would have been just my limited
and superficial thoughts and assumptions.

I can see that my whole life has been a training to reach this
point. I was born to two very mild-mannered parents, which is an
essential quality of a yogi. I went through the first ten years of life
being grounded and rooted by these souls, who lived in a peaceful
way. Another important part of a yogic upbringing is my early experience with separation. Being separated from my family for some
years helped me develop a kind of detachment and independence
that yogis need.

I joined the beauty world and traveled the globe, being exposed
to things in the outer world to the point where I had very few desires left. This exposure to people around the world gave me an
acceptance of all beings no matter their color, sexuality, or actions.

I was mentored in natural medicine and spirituality starting at
nineteen, so while I was living the path of outer beauty to the fullest, I was also being taught the fundamentals of inner beauty. With
hindsight, I can now see that I went through the perfect training
and journey to where I am today.

Take a moment to look over your life's journey and see where
you are and what the meaning of all your experiences has been. You
will probably surprise yourself to learn how you got where you are
today and what that means.

Discovering Your Dharma

If you were born in the Western culture or lifestyle, chances are as a youngster you were encouraged to ask questions so you could learn more and become smarter. At school you asked even more questions in order to decipher complex formulas and complicated equations. You were told to focus on your homework, study, and get ready to make a living. This is when you developed most of your ideas of who you would become in this world.

Then after all the questioning comes another period of your life when you go from asking to telling. As we become older we feel we know enough, so we start to tell people what we think and feel. We share our opinions freely on just about everything, even when we don't know what we are talking about (or even when people haven't asked for our opinion). This phase starts the *me* period. It's the time when not much else matters except our own needs and wants. Anyone or anything that can fulfill our desires is pretty much what we are interested in at this stage. It's when we want validation and acceptance, and we will find it anywhere we can.

But as children and into adolescence, if we were introduced to the concept and philosophy of *dharma*, or life principles or purpose, we would learn not to put so much attention on our mind self and instead put more on the bigger picture of our life in a community. Shifting our attention to the global community does two things: it stabilizes the mind from any stress of competition, and it helps a developing brain always to think in terms of a bigger collective community and inclusivity of everyone.

In other words, it doesn't allow for separateness, and this inclusivity always makes our mind feel supported. Instead of asking "Why can't I have . . ." or "When am I going to get . . ." we should be teaching our young ones to ask and contemplate: "Who am I and what is my purpose?" These questions would set in motion a great life of searching for, finding, and living out our destiny on a conscious level where fulfillment of the soul and mind can be the result. This would bring great inner contentment and relieve people's pursuit of an unattainable and temporary happiness for the rest of their life.

We are usually too immature to understand what our purpose means even as adults, unless we have been brought up in a Buddhist or Hindu household or follow a path that believes in dharma and the journey of the soul from past lives. It takes an evolved soul to ask a mature question like: "What is my purpose and reason for existing in this body?" This evolved questioning is usually undertaken by a soul who has come from a past life of spiritual grounding and higher consciousness.

Although this is a question everyone should be asking themselves, it probably only enters a few people's mind once in a while as a passing thought or in a casual conversation. This is because this question needs many years of contemplation and searching before arriving at a conclusive answer.

Very few minds recognize their soul's purpose in a lifetime; most are more interested and focused on their mind's journey of creative discoveries and expression. I once asked one of the most famous technological geniuses of our generation what his purpose was, and he replied with a distant look, "That's a great question." He looked at me as if I had just asked him to remember what he had eaten on his fourth birthday at exactly 2:37 in the afternoon. In other words, he was stumped because he had spent little or no time contemplating this question. He might have thought because he was a huge inventor and wealthy man that everything to be discovered was on the outside. Interestingly enough, fifteen minutes into the conversation, I also discovered he didn't have much drive to do anything else now that he had made such a massive impact on society and become wealthy to the point he could buy anything; he didn't know how to top what he had achieved outwardly. This is, after all, the limit of the mind: it can speak, build, and gather, but it can't lead us to higher levels like fulfillment and self-realization.

The outer world is so tangible that most minds don't even see the point in thinking about something so out of reach as looking inward. But not pursuing our purpose is like being a singer who has been offered a five-album deal but instead chooses to get drunk and ends up never recording a song. Not pursuing our purpose will leave a hole in our heart and be very disappointing because we have not achieved our ultimate goal in life.

There are many purposes that bring our soul into this body we live in. There is always the one overall bigger purpose that runs through our entire life, but then there are also many smaller purposeful events and journeys that we have to go through that are all a part of the same greater purpose. The challenge we are presented with is to know what our purpose is, be it big or small, long term or short term. The even bigger challenge is to know if it is our soul's purpose we are following or whether our mind has made up something to fulfill and is now taking us on a whirlwind journey of outer pursuits.

Are You Following Mind or Spirit Dharma?

Our one and only purpose as a soul traveler is liberation—liberation from the physical body and liberation from the material plane. And liberation comes once we have achieved our life purpose and fulfilled dharma during this lifespan. So we have one purpose to live for and one to die for. To be able to fulfill our life purpose is to complete our time in a human body and to move on to higher dimensions, such as *anandamaya kosha*, the blissful spiritual state one step above our intellect. For this we need dharma to help us on the journey.

Dharma has many definitions, from Buddhist teachings to the Rig Veda, an ancient collection of Vedic Sanskrit hymns. It means the energy that is part of the cosmic order. It means behavior, a right way of living according to ancient texts. But what dharma mainly helps us do is live out our purpose.

It is a road map for our behavior and conduct that helps keep us on course toward our spiritual goals. It is also what deters us from all outward distractions that the world presents us with on a daily basis. It sets out our duties and creates order on a personal, individual level as well as on a grander community plane. As our soul or higher Self has come into the world and taken up this body to fulfill specific goals, some rules of conduct need to be followed for our mind not to be distracted and lost in the outer world.

But as we can observe in our own life and the people around us, our mind has taken control of the body and kidnapped it away from the spirit. It has taken control and is in the pursuit of all things outward. All the things like entertainment, pleasure, and happiness have become more important; these are all outer material and emotional distractions from our original spiritual purpose. Although they don't lead us anywhere in particular, this pursuit seems much more attractive than trying to live a purposeful life that seems rigid and one we didn't choose. It's like the reality of not being able to choose your family members but having the choice of which friends to have in your life and for how long.

Our modern society has been built on business and negotiations, so the evidence of ego identity is everywhere for us to observe. This is a very "normal" way of building a life out of a material existence, and everything around us supports this way of living. Every aspect of our life—food, conversations, work, family, relationships—has become entwined with artificial products in artificial environments. Our sense of what is real and what is not has become very confused and distorted. This is what the mind purpose does—it confuses itself into thinking it needs to take control of the outer nature instead of controlling itself.

An example of this is the way we refer to food. Food used to be just called food. Then we started to use chemical pesticides and had to start to differentiate between organic and nonorganic food. Then once we began to genetically engineer food, we had to differentiate between organic, nonorganic, and genetically modified food (GMO). Nature provides the most perfect and natural necessities for our existence, and the mind finds a way to justify the need to alter it and make it "better." This is an example of a mind pursuit and not a spiritual purpose being fulfilled. The mind's standards are very low, while the soul's purpose is the pursuit of spiritual perfection. We are pursuing perfection of our minds through science and medicine, trying to live as long as possible and look as young as science allows. The fear of getting old and dying has become our biggest distraction from fulfilling dharma, while dying purposefully should be one of our higher pursuits.

Our dharma or purpose as yogis isn't to try and live as long as possible but to live out our purpose and then to know the exact second we should let go of the physical body. This is the sign that our purpose has been completed. This is truly living without fear and living with spiritual purpose. This is the most liberating way to exist.

For instance, the death of a six-month-old child or someone having an unfortunate accident is not just coincidence or bad luck. There is a timer on each one of our bodies that is counting down without our awareness. Yes, you can step in front of a bus and end your life seemingly whenever you want, but even that event is predetermined because of past karmas. Karma is not limited to one lifetime. To live the yogic life brings you to this awareness.

We have come from another life, and our destiny is to pass through and continue on to the next level. When the body expires it is time for the spirit to move on, as its purpose has been fulfilled in this particular body. If we focus on our life from this point of view, all of the fears and confusion we have collected in our mind will disappear and we will be much more conscious of our higher dharma.

Dharmic Living Practices

So what is dharmic living and how do we follow it? There are many practices of dharmic living, but few that people in ordinary life can follow without getting lost or being discouraged by them. Life is moving fast, and people want to get on with living without having to spend too much time on discipline or self-control. These topics are considered boring and time consuming. But without them the heart never becomes open and content. What is useful for us is not to change the practices or follow watered-down versions or pieces of the practices, but to bring in the ones that are most relevant to our lifestyle now and practice them fully. This way we can use them and be encouraged by our progress, knowing we are still practicing an authentic practice and at a manageable level. Through this encouragement we will have the natural urge to keep building on our progress as we see what amazing effects they have on our mind and body.

If dharma is the road map and the purpose is the goal, the journey needs to be planned out. This is not so much to avoid pitfalls as to be able to manage them when they occur. With this approach we don't quickly become discouraged or disillusioned by life as it brings with it all the surprises that it has in store for us to live fully.

Dharmic living tools are what we need for our mind to grasp its duties and purposeful living standards along this journey of life we are taking. These dharmic practices are like the green and red lights of traffic signals, letting us know when it is appropriate to move and when it is time to stop. They are the protective barriers and railings as you drive along mountainous roads. They are the gas and brake pedals of your enthusiasm and your fears. They are what conserve your energy and teach you how and when to use it. Without this directive our minds don't know how to interact with others in a peaceful and purposeful manner. We also won't know our limits and boundaries.

Dharma is not for limiting our lives but, on the contrary, to assist us in living them fully. It helps to create safety barriers from the outer world taking over our minds and harming our bodies. These practices were put in place by ancient seers to help each one of us reach our individual greatness. When we keep a more disciplined and aware manner of living, our inner potential comes shining through. Like when you repeat a mantra for the first time and you start to feel its energy opening up inside. As you keep repeating it over and over the vibration reverberates around your whole being and keeps revealing more of your inner dimensions that were hidden before.

This is the concept of a secret. A secret is information that we are not aware of yet. If someone tells us something we don't know, it becomes apparent only on an intellectual level. So if I tell you the mantra *om* is the universal sound of the cosmic consciousness, you will take that as information. If you start to repeat it, then it becomes a practical exercise. If you start to practice it every day as part of you spiritual routine, over time you will experience the infinite expanse of it within you. And if you continue this for the rest of your life, you will be at one with the cosmic consciousness that once was just information or a secret to your mind.

This is how we follow the yogic path, because in it is contained all the universal secrets. We practice, and the rest just happens from inside, revealing itself the more you do your practice. Yoga is actually what is inside of you and not what anyone can teach you or give to you. True yoga is the unveiling of your spiritual Self and the uniting of it with the universal energy through *moksha*, or liberation.

PRACTICE PEACEFULNESS

The first and most important dharmic practice is nonviolence. I say most important because of the violent and conflicted times we exist in. We are not just at war with others, we are in a constant conflict with ourselves and the planet through our manner of living. Without attention to nonviolence and peace, finding and living out our purpose is very difficult. Violence is physical, mental, and spiritual, just like anything else. The physical pain we inflict on another living organism is eventually felt by all living beings around the globe, as we are all connected. When we inflict mental shame on ourselves, we are creating inharmonious vibrations that are damaging to every cell of our body and mind, changing our thought patterns and emotional stability. This inner vibrational energy is also felt by every living being, although we might feel we are keeping it to ourselves and no one else knows about it or can feel it. We are one large, pulsating cell that seems individual on the limited outer level but which is actually part of a whole particle on an inner dimension. That's why one person's pain is a collective pain, why one's contentment is everyone's joy.

The idea "I am bad, sad, angry, or just not good enough" carries with it energy that depletes the body and mind. It takes energy away from them and creates *dis*ease, as does the energy of "I am the best, I'm amazing, I'm better than you," which is the extreme of the former that weakens our divine vibration, bringing us lower into a place of mind conflict. The body and mind are just vibrations. And vibrations change direction, amplify, or lower depending on the one who is controlling the volume. It's easy to say to you, "Don't be harmful to yourself or others." It's another thing to be able to do this when you need to practice this form of dharma. The trick is not to wait until the occasion demands it but to practice at all times. This way we will be in a nonviolent habit, so when a challenging moment arises that needs more effort, we have the practice to rise above it.

Once you start to recognize and identify your biggest triggers of violent behavior, you can either avoid certain people and situations until you have more practice being peaceful or practice detachment in the moment so the energy of the situation doesn't affect you as much. If you have a friend who loves to eat and drink a lot, for example, and you recognize it as a violent pattern harmful to the body and mind that you also follow, then you might avoid that friend until you feel stronger, more able to say no to excessive consuming. Or if you have a family member you can't avoid who seems to always say something in your presence to upset you, practicing patience and detachment would be necessary to get you through the moment with them. Your approach to nonviolence should always be peaceful, but not with an expectation that others will reciprocate the same energy.

PRACTICE CREATIVE CONTROL

The second dharmic practice is to control our sexual energy. This has become one of the most confusing and frustrating aspects of our society, and anything that is this distracting and misused will pull us away further from our purpose. As most people consider sex and sexuality to be a very natural feeling, they are not sure why it needs controlling. Is sex mainly for pleasure and fulfilling our lustful and love desires, or is it meant for conserving and using for other creative endeavors like procreation? This energy is the most powerful and prominent force in our society.

Everything around us is controlled or directed by sexual energy. It's not just in the obvious moments when you see a naked person or receive a sensual touch. It runs much deeper than this. For instance, watch your next few TV commercials with an eye to how you are sold a product. It is either through fear or sexual power. It's called "empowering" you! It's everywhere we look and listen. We are told we are in control because we can choose one thing over another or one person over another. We are taught to succeed and push ourselves at work, in relationships, and at the gym. All this is the accumulation and use of sexual energy.

Everything we are trying to do takes energy, and this is all sexual energy, because it all originates in the lower chakra, or energy point, that controls the genitals.

When this energy stays in the lower regions of the body it is mainly used for physical and material desires, but when moved upward through the yogic practices I outline in the practice chapter, this energy gathers momentum and becomes very subtle and much more powerful, moving into the heart or anahata chakra. This is when our mind focuses more on our ultimate purpose and leaves the surface indulgences aside. Most people never move out of the surface life dramas of the mind and issues of the body because they are focused on outer pleasures and desires through food, relationships, and sex. The senses are fully in control of a person's mind, so the outer world seems very real and the mind is invested in all activities and emotional feelings of day-to-day life.

When you start to follow a more yogic life and routine you allow for this sexual energy to become controlled, creative, and directed at will. As it rises up further through all the chakras, your ideas and drive become focused more on spiritual matters and less on fulfilling the ego desires of the body or mind. You start to spend more time fulfilling the divine's purpose, which is coming through the body and focusing less on what the mind thinks is important. Sometimes you hear stories of wandering *sadhus*, or mendicants, in India who came from rich families but gave up everything to live a life of solitude and discipline. They don't want anything and they don't own anything. But notably they are always ready to serve and have this inner glow or contentment within. Anytime I have met such beings, they all say the same thing: once they were directed by their heart or inner divine nature, it became unproductive for them to live as a regular person as they had before.

We are sometimes misguided by professionals in our modern society who teach that lots of sex is great for health and our relationships, but then we live in a society of frustrated people who are having sex, in some cases with many people, while few seem to be satisfied or fulfilled mentally or spiritually. It is not a case of sex is good or bad but more an individual decision about how best to use this energy for maximum satisfaction. This really becomes a personal choice about how to use this powerful energy. We have such potent energy at our disposal that has the power to heal and deliver most of our goals to us, and if we learn how to apply it in the yogic way, we will move past all frustrations and start to live with maximum potency and vigor for life.

We don't use this energy to its fullest potential because of a lack of discipline, or maybe because we haven't thought about how else to use it. But it's like having the energy of lightning at our disposal and merely using it to light a candle.

PRACTICE LESS IS MORE

The third dharmic practice is to avoid burdensome excesses. This is basically the concept of not taking or consuming more than we need. How much is too much and how much makes us greedy? Again, this is a very individual amount, but it's less about quantity and more about why we need something in the first place. Are things that we desire necessities or our endless wants? Our desires have grown so much that they are pulling us far away from our purpose. Most of our so-called needs are really the mind justifying why it can't live without something or someone.

For sadhus, who give up everything and live with just the clothes on their back, it's not that there are not enough clothes in the world, but rather they don't need more than they have. A person who buys two homes is called a good investor in our society, but it is this action that drives up the price of houses and leaves others behind to suffer, for they cannot even afford one house. Greed is not a matter of morals or economics; it's a matter of asking the question, do we need more?

But greed doesn't need to be physical to harm us. For example, when we take in too much information it is very distracting to the mind. When it is an overload for our brain, it becomes disturbing.

We've become information junkies. People are collecting information and storing it for the future, not realizing that we need
knowledge and experience, because information alone is not of
any use to us on our higher quest for our purpose. But much of
the information we are collecting is mostly without our conscious
awareness. It is sensory greed. And this sensory greed is insatiable
if left uncontrolled. The reason we have sense control exercises in
our spiritual practice is exactly to curb this overload.

Excess takes on many other forms in the context of emotions,
time, money, food, attention seeking, fame, material objects, and
so on. We are all acquisitive in one way or another, and it takes a
balanced mind to understand how much and when is enough. A
simple rule of practice can be first to contemplate and wait before
making a decision. This pause will give you the opportunity to
see what other thoughts come into play. Yesterday, for example,
I wanted to store some documents on a portable hard drive. I'd
dropped the one I had, and it broke. So I went looking in a few
boxes for an old drive but didn't find one. Then I went on the
Internet to order one, but before pressing Buy, I decided to make
a cup of tea. I remembered my social media guys telling me they
store everything online. Then I realized I already had this service,
which I was using for photos and videos. In a matter of minutes
I went from buying something I didn't need to using something I
already had.

This is a small example but relevant to the subject at hand. In my own life, I search for reasons why I shouldn't consume more rather than talk myself into buying what I don't need. I test my judgments or decisions to consume more based on simple truths. Will acquiring more of something add to my life? Will it be excessive to do so? Is consumption harmonious with the lifestyle I have chosen? This approach makes life so much simpler and takes all the doubt or temptations away quickly. With this approach we will only consume exactly what is necessary and cut out a lot of unneeded collecting of stuff, be it material or mental.

On our path to our purpose and living out that purpose, we need as few distractions as possible and as much discipline and control of our senses and mind as possible. The outer world is not much help to us in this regard, because everything around us is constantly drawing us outward to consume more. The yogic practices are here to assist us in keeping on this path of simplicity so we don't forget our purpose, which is easy to do. This way we can fulfill our dharma and live a purposeful life.

Chapter Summary

- Are you living your mind's purpose or your soul's purpose?
- The mind makes up and changes purposes regularly. The Self directs us to the same purposes.

- ◆ What is your ultimate purpose?
- ◆ Follow the three dharmic practices to be able to exert more self-control and self-discipline and ultimately arrive at your purpose.

Daily Life Practice

In doing the three dharmic practices, you will find great strength and discipline to move closer to uncovering your ultimate purpose, and they will also guide you to live with more awareness and higher knowledge so you can fulfill your purpose.

Knowing your purpose is one part of the puzzle. It's like having the correct map to the right destination. The other half is to have the expertise through yogic practices to live it and reach the ultimate destination without fear or hesitation and above all without being distracted by life.

1. Peacefulness comes as a result of letting go of conflicts. I personally avoid conflicts by repeating the words: "It's just mind stuff." This way no matter who says what, I know it is just their mind saying stuff and not a reflection of their pure soul. Just repeating these few words internally will help you not take anything personally or react to other people's words.

2. Control of our creative energy is essential for our health as well as for our focus. It's how we retain our power. The energy of prana is also in this force. I put most of my sexual, creative energy into practice, purpose, and relationships. The more you put your energy into meaningful actions that use up this power, the more this power will come back to energize you. Some of it used for physical pleasure is a wonderful experience, but storing up and using this energy on your spiritual life will make the energy even more potent for you to reach all your goals and feel fulfilled on the physical, mental, and spiritual levels.

3. Practicing less is more is basically about turning your eyes, ears, and touch away from things you want more of. Everyone has vices and things that get their attention. In our household, we have decided to live with as few things as possible so we can put most of our attention on what matters to us and not in having to take care and preserve what we own. If what you own starts to own you, then it is time to let go of some things.

Service: The Key to Empowerment

On one of our recent trips to India, Jaimyse and I went to Rikhia-peeth ashram in north India to train in a particular form of tantric practice. Swami Satyasangananda Saraswati, who is the direct disciple of Swami Satyananda Saraswati from the Sivananda lineage, was teaching the *Soundarya Lahari*, a famous literary tantric work in Sanskrit. Its beautiful and powerful teachings include the practices of mantra with focus on the chakras while using *yantras* (meditative geometrical shapes). If you can master these practices you can master your many life journeys. You come to learn that giving is empowering.

During and after our training each day, we also had to do *seva*, or selfless service. We were assigned duties of either packing rice or wrapping packages for the villagers. Many of the villagers who come to the ashram are widows who have nowhere to go and no one to help them except for the ashram.

Seva is done with no agenda, wants, likes, or conditions. It's a training in giving and being of service, an attitude of giving time and energy for the good of others. It's a rather simple practice to perform in the ashram when everyone around is involved in it, but may not be such a simple or practical practice on the outside. On one of our breaks from seva, I was telling Jaima that I remember doing a lot of this work during my travels and visits to different ashrams over the years. I was commenting that it would be so easy for me to live in an ashram and submit to this way of living, but I didn't feel that seva was a big part of my present daily path right now, especially back at home away from the ashram.

This led me to wonder why I wasn't bringing seva into my life and work in a greater way all the time. I certainly recognized that the way I gave my service in an ashram, asking people where I could help next, was not my normal way of living at home. My excuse was that at home I am far too busy working and don't have time. But what about an attitude of being of service, do I have that? Honestly, the answer is a yes and a no.

The next day we had a one-on-one with Swami Satyasanga-nanda to ask questions and seek guidance on different parts of life. As she was speaking, one thing stood out from everything else she said: "The underlying teachings that Sri Guru Satyananda and this ashram are teaching is seva. All the other practices are a support to this. Seva is the true practice of yoga, as it breaks down all barriers of the mind, importance, and ideas standing in the way of reaching the spirit of love."

There are no coincidences. I had to hear this message, and in contemplating it, I saw that I was being challenged to go deeper in my service. I had to examine and make decisions on how to integrate seva into my daily life at home, especially when it can feel challenging. I realized that at home I needed to find a balance between my work life and my private life, otherwise I would not be able to sustain either one.

But most important, what I learned from Swamiji (the suffix *-ji* is an honorific used as a term of respect in India) was that how we approach our work and life as a service to humanity matters more, and we should always be open to everyone. Although I spend a lot of my time consulting with clients, at workshops with students, or writing material for people to improve their lives, I still don't always feel fully in service to others, as some people invariably are left behind. But after all, nothing is perfect, is it?

Selfless Service

Different centuries and ages have gone through their own challenges based on the collective karmas that had to be worked through at that time. There are four *yugas* (eras) mentioned in the yogic texts. Sat Yuga is the lightest and most conscious age, when people act out of love and the higher Self, while Kali Yuga is the exact opposite. You could say Kali Yuga is the age of ego and mind, while Sat Yuga is the age of bliss and divine existence. In the time of Kali Yuga, which we are now passing through or have come to the end of (various scholars mark the timing differently), the energy of this age is much heavier than all other times.

I think everyone is feeling the effects of this yuga or the remnants of its energy in a big way; it's impossible to get away from or remain unaffected by it. With the denseness of this yuga come manifestations and the strong tendency toward materialism and extreme consumption, so we are all challenged to keep our minds calm and in control. This makes it very difficult for us to act out of pure love and selflessness because the mind's nature is preoccupied with personal wants. "Taking care of number one" is one description of our age that is very appropriate.

This age makes it virtually impossible to act in true service to another, but at the same time it is service that we need to help us connect with each other—making someone or something else more important. Mothers usually have this gift naturally when their baby is born or they are looking after a sick child. The nurturing feminine energy feels for others much quicker than the fiery male energy does. Fighters and conquerors are typically men or women with a lot of masculine energy. The female energy wants to heal and take care of others, while the masculine energy wants to fight and control. But only an individual truly balanced in both male and female energy can serve others in a complete manner.

A person with excessive feminine energy can become too smothering in their nature, acting out of their fear of what will happen to the other person if they don't help them. Or a person with too much masculine energy can have a hardness and pushiness where they feel they know best and all the other person needs to do is obey. True service requires us to first be balanced in our own thoughts and actions before we start to help others. Otherwise we will bring even more imbalance to an already imbalanced situation instead of assisting it. Service to others deflates the ego mind and allows the heart to speak and act. It takes all the thinking out of the scenario and allows for communion of hearts.

Pure service is giving without any expectations or the urge to receive in return. It is selfless in body, mind, and spirit. The actual receiving comes as a by-product of giving. It is payback in karma currency, which has endless positive energy. And with this payback the energy is not just for the doer, but for all mankind. It is like an investment made in the name of all beings. This is not giving to charity because we get a tax deduction or because we feel we should help once in a while. It is not helping someone because it makes us feel good or because we feel bad for them. It is not giving out of guilt or out of fear. It is putting everyone first and ourselves last.

Real service goes beyond mutual needs or everyday give-and-take. Most of us understand service as giving but not as a state of being. When giving to charity, we exchange money for a feeling of being part of something. It is a momentary service but not a mind-set of being of service to humanity on a continuous basis. It is selective service.

True seva requires us to be of service at any time and for anyone or anything. Seva is not a selective process to a truly giving person. The openness of giving is a state of mind rather than of a physical nature. We can't be in multiple places at the same time, so we can only serve where we are in a physical way. But we are also only useful in certain situations and to certain people. Because we have free time doesn't mean that we are running around trying to give or assist others to fill time.

Late one evening, Jaima (my wife's spiritual name) was sitting in our Brahmin brother Suresh's home in the village where we live in India when a man walked in. I was not there, but Jaima recounted the story to me the next day. It seemed more likely than not this man had been drinking alcohol. Now, you don't find many people who drink around the temple, as no shops sell alcohol. Sometimes people pick it up at someone's house on their travels, but in the village no one openly drinks, as it is not part of the custom.

When the man started asking Jaima for water she went to get Manjunath, one of the occupants of the house. He came out and saw the man was somewhat tipsy. He gave the man some water but didn't ask him to leave. Then fifteen minutes later, Suresh came in and started talking to Jaima. She brought his attention to the drunk man in the corner. Suresh went to the man and asked him what he needed. The man needed a place to stay for the night. So Suresh went and cleared out the front room of some bags and showed the man to his room.

Suresh, already knowing what Jaima was thinking, said, "Guests are God. The divine is in all of us no matter what we are putting in our bodies, and in turning away the man we would be turning away the divine herself." True service is not prejudiced and it doesn't pass judgment. True service is not about giving and not receiving. It's just about doing for others as they need and not always what we think they need.

Then we can also be of service mentally and spiritually by praying, contemplating, or thinking of others. Here is where each of the sacred rituals in this book are connected and support one another. When we perform our daily spiritual practice and find our purpose, we then make service our natural progression from these two rituals. No matter what job we have, we can bring the attitude of service into it rather than thinking what we can get out of it. If I am traveling to a place where there is a smaller audience, I don't think I have to make less effort because the numbers are smaller and it is less important to offer them my best energy. On the contrary, it is a great opportunity to give people an even better personal experience.

Thus our work becomes a matter of not what we can get but

what kind of service we can offer. Bringing the attitude of seva into your job is to do it for the love of the people and the work. It is connecting to others beyond just the physical nature and more on the spiritual level. For example, in the service industry you are used to being there to assist and make people's lives simpler by providing them with your service. This practice may resonate with you much more than, say, someone who is working to pick food on a farm. Although picking fruits and vegetables may be more of an indirect service, nevertheless it is a very necessary part of serving one another.

But even then we could go further and recognize that without Mother Nature providing the seed, soil, rain, and sun nothing would grow for anyone to pick or consume. So it starts with Mother Nature showing the way as an example of selflessness and service by providing our essential necessities and it ends up in our hands to continue the same state of being with all other living creatures.

Of course, if you want to go further into the attitude and practice of service on an even deeper individual level, you will contemplate the work you do and the effects of it on all beings and the environment. Does your vocation support companies and brands that put toxins into the environment? Or does your work include producing foods and drinks that destroy people's health? When you want to go deeper with your service-oriented life, you will come across many obstacles in your way that challenge the nature of your habits, work, and beliefs. This is where your true intentions will be challenged to show themselves.

Being of service is not always a straightforward choice. This is why you first need to know your motivations for what you do. If, for example, you go out to get just any job or to do any kind of work just to make money, you won't be necessarily fulfilling your purpose, and you may also not be feeling that you are of service to others. Life is a domino effect of events and choices, their reactions, and our reactions to the reactions. This is how karma is created and lived out by us and through us. We are walking and talking karma machines. Everything has a reaction and repercussion on some level for us all.

The other thing with seva is that although we have an attitude of service to all, it doesn't mean that we run ourselves into the ground trying to attend to everyone, because that would not be helpful on a bigger scale. We should first become focused in our practice and purpose, so when the opportunity arises to be of service, we know exactly if we should get involved and to what degree. There still needs to be a balance even when serving.

We want to be of service to the people we are best suited to serve and events in which we can be used in the best possible way. We are all skilled in different ways, so our service needs to be focused in areas where we can make the biggest impact—in terms not of numbers but of efficiency. There is an art to this, which becomes evident once we get to know ourselves better through self-study.

Service Is Different from Helping

Our society views the concept of helping as a way of expressing our selflessness. People are constantly using the words *helping*, *sacrificing*, or *giving up*, which denotes that someone can't or won't help themselves. Helping another is more of an ego mind concept than actual service. This is why people have so many conflicts with others and say, "I was only trying to help." Many people think I can help them. I have never helped anyone in reality. I have guided others to help themselves through changes they have decided to make. They took the action, not me. My work is more to shine a light on people's inner strength, knowledge, and power that most have forgotten about or lost the ability to use at will.

My guru, for instance, never helped me with anything either. He gave me instructions, he showed me the practices and shared the knowledge, but then he left me to practice while looking over me to make sure I was following the correct instructions. So all one can actually do is give us the manual, describe the process, and provide the tools. We become weaker when someone tries to help us by doing what we should be doing.

There are so many examples of this in our society. When a baby is learning to stand and keeps falling, the parents usually help it up. If you catch the flu, your doctor usually prescribes medication to help relieve the symptoms, but this weakens your body's immune system instead of allowing it to fight off the virus and become stronger. I have a client who talks to her friend in another country two or three times a day for a few hours at a time, listening to her suffering and pain. My client has now become the crutch and obstacle, not the solution to her friend's issues. There are many more examples of so-called helping. We might think something or someone is helping us, but actually in the long run they are undermining our strength, which needs to find its way out through experience. The solution is in the practice, action, and experience, not in the help we get to avoid our issues.

Some will ask what about feeding the poor, the sick, and the elderly? What about charity and giving? What about research to cure diseases and provide homes for the abused? Isn't that helping people, as they can't help themselves? It is the mind that thinks they can't help themselves. It is also the mind that wants to control the situation because it feels it has the answers to other people's issues. It's not to say that people don't need some assistance, but only to the degree that it helps them help themselves and not to the degree our mind thinks they need help. Everyone needs to live out their karma, otherwise they will have to continue going through the same issues over and over until they work through them.

Our concept of giving and being of service basically comes down to helping people for a day here or there because it is a holiday or to sending them some money. We give billions to charity, to cure cancer, or to vaccinate a whole continent. These impulses may have all the right intentions behind them, but tend to produce a different effect or outcome from what might be intended. We have the same attitude to service as we do with modern medicine. Put a bandage on the problem and only treat the symptom. We are not helping the solution but perpetuating more symptoms.

True service is an attitude that we bring into our actions and not just the action itself.

When I went to Cambodia to teach young girls who had been sexually abused and trafficked, I never felt that they needed my help as I didn't see them as victims. Or when I was invited to Afghanistan to teach meditation to soldiers and inmates, I didn't see myself as a helper. I was just there sharing some time with other beings. I hope what they got from it was equal to what I did: a beautiful experience of interaction, laughter, and a lot of emotional and mental healing, which they really needed. I got to experience a fraction of their pain and

100 percent of their joy. It was not really an equal exchange from my point of view.

We are now going through many climate changes and environmental challenges, so another popular movement is to "help" the planet. How can we help a planet? A planet is a living organism that has an immune system much stronger than ours. Mother Nature is constantly cleaning herself, and when needed, she will, through the help of other planets, do her inner cleansing of people and our destructive ways. So yes, we are polluting the earth at a rapid pace, but she doesn't need our help. If anything, we need her help to not become extinct.

What we need is not to help the planet, but to be of service to it by curbing our individual and collective toxic lifestyles of excessive consumption and using more than we need. If we lived with the minimum we need instead of the excess we want, everyone would be content and we wouldn't be polluting the atmosphere, water, and land. After all, we can't be excessive and help the planet at the same time.

There is a very fine line between the ego mind helping and the spirit guiding us to be of service without disturbing another being's karmic journey. One comes from our "common sense" or our own fears, while the other comes out of direct divine intervention. The outcome of our directive from our higher Self isn't always understood by the mind because it isn't logical or something the mind wants to do. Because our higher Self comes from a limitless and fearless place, it usually scares the mind, as the mind feels lost and out of control. This becomes confusing to us, as we want to always feel in control.

Spirituality and acting out of soul consciousness is not after all an intellectual process.

Being of Real Service

Being of true service is to act out of our heart's spirit in a selfless way and put the other person first no matter who they are and what they have done. It is not to pick and choose based on good or bad or our preference. When we act out of selfless service, there are no prejudices in our mind as to why one deserves our attention and another doesn't. In fact, when we give to a person or cause that we don't agree with but know it is of great value to everyone, it can be a much bigger act of giving than one we are committed to, which is easier. This is why it is not easy to be of pure service, because our minds are full of likes and dislikes based on personal and collective preconceptions and prejudices.

If we want to serve others on the purest level we first need to serve our spirit/soul. Our spirit is our inner guru and guide. It is our intuition and goes much deeper and beyond our limited mind. To start to become a selfless being we have to first tame the senses and mind that are the causes of our self-centeredness. Our body needs to be as pure as possible and our mind as focused as neces-sary. This needs to happen through keeping our diet balanced, our conversations purposeful, our ears away from harmful sounds, our mind away from unnecessary thoughts, and our eyes away from temptations as we keep our touch only for things that serve our path.

If we follow the yogic practices and first learn to serve our inner teacher, then we will be directed from within by our intuition, not just to be of service but for all things in our life. It will remove the fear and limited thoughts of the mind, which are placing doubt on the situation. You will see as you cultivate this ritual along this journey that many revelations start to unfold.

When we start to make our inner guru and others our focus and not just ourselves, our interests, our work, our cause, and so on will suddenly start to shift and we will notice everything in a whole new light. We start to notice others on a deeper level with-out placing any limitations of color, sexuality, or religion on them. We pay more attention to others, not just listening to what they are saying but seeing ourselves in them. This is where we start to break down the walls of separation and enter the vastness and expanse of unity through a limitless mind.

Once you see others as yourself, then by serving them you are also serving yourself and your inner Self. This becomes the genu-ine and complete circle of service while being served.

Chapter Summary

- Being of service is thinking of others before yourself.
- It isn't always clear when we are being of service or a hindrance, which is why we need inner guidance.
- Giving people what they want and not what we want to give is being of service to them.
- Selfless service is an essential part of walking the yogic path and creating a balance in society.

Daily Life Practice

1. Look at your life and see how you spend most of your time each day. Is there a part of your day when you are being of service, and if so, can you be more present? Are you giving more importance to your cell phone, social media, or work when you should be listening to a loved one or someone in need?

2. Each week, make sure to do a few things during the day for others, and build on this. For instance, one of the ways I serve others is by spending time outside of my work schedule answering their questions about their health issues or giving spiritual guidance about their practice. What you decide to do should have the atti-

tude of service in it, and it can be as much or as little as you choose.

3. Be of service to humanity also by expanding your mind and letting go of some of the prejudices you have acquired. This could be a dislike toward a person or group for what they stand for. It could be toward other countries or religions. In being of service, we don't need to go to war to serve but to control the wars in our mind that we burden other people with.

8

Love: The Key to Everyone's Heart

The village in south India that Jaima and I live in part of the year has a temple dedicated to Devi, a female goddess who is the embodiment of femininity and love. People come there to be in her presence because of the *shakti,* or feminine energy, she emanates.

The sage Shankaracharya had seen a vision in the forest some fourteen hundred years before and placed Mookambika, or "Mother," as she is known, in the temple surrounded by tigers and cobras. Her figure sits in the center of the small temple within the inner sanctum that only a handful of Brahmins (priests) can enter. There are many rituals that are performed before her, which are done daily for people who come to worship and be in her energy.

One day we were sitting with our spiritual brother Shreesha, whose family has been watching over and taking care of the goddess for the last few hundred years. He is one of the few who is allowed to bathe and touch the deity. Shreesha was telling us the story of the first time he stepped into the inner sanctum, when his father and grandfather took care of Mookambika, and how it became his turn to start looking after her when he was a young man.

He told us that no one could prepare him for entering that small room in the temple. His father never discussed it, because it is something you need to go through without the mind being involved. When he stepped into the chamber, he could barely stand and was falling to his knees. The energy of the deity was so intense that the normal, physical body couldn't withstand it. His body was vibrating so much he had to step back outside for a minute. As he was recounting this experience, his eyes became very intense, and after a pause, he said, "The energy of love is so strong that I couldn't withstand it in my body."

Since visiting this temple and meditating there for a few years now, I know what he is speaking about, but not with that kind of intensity. I can only imagine how immense that energy must have been for my friend Shreesha, because the energy is still very intense sitting some distance away outside of the inner sanctum. Love is truly in the air.

The Source of All Love

Love is called and described in so many different ways. It is elusive but so desired by everyone. It is harsh but so sweet. It is painful but so necessary. It is the one thing all beings crave but find difficult to get enough of or keep. There is no other topic more spoken, written, sung, or painted about than love. It is the silent and invisible energy at the heart of every person's desires and passion. It is also the most misunderstood and unattained experience at the highest level.

But this is all the mind's idea of love and not love itself. Ideology is not truth or universal reality. It is a limited and compartmentalized idea based on our upbringing and what we believe. There is so much unnecessary suffering going on between people in all kinds of friendships and relationships due to the misperception of what love is and isn't. We all have too many misguided expectations of what it should be according to our desires. Love is not a feeling but a knowing and being. Feelings come from the mind and senses. Knowing comes from our intuition and heart center—namely the seat of the divine. Our body is the lighthouse, and the beacon is the seat of the Self, shining from inward. Because our attention is on the outer world through our interactions, we are constantly being pulled outward to experience love on a very surface level. We are constantly surfing the waves of love but never diving into the endless depths of it.

No one can experience the purest of love, which is untainted by the mind, unless we turn our attention inward and plug into this divine energy. This is actually only the first step. The effort of moving our attention from outer to inner through the yogic practices discussed in this book is the groundwork for the next stage. These practices are the tools necessary to unveil love. Once we have practiced for a long time and without interruption, pure love becomes a reality not by searching for or attaining it but by becoming and dissolving into it. It's when the mind is no longer in the way. Like a curtain that has been drawn back to show what is behind it, when we draw the curtain of the mind all the way back, we will then unveil our true divine nature of love.

In this sense the mind can't experience pure love, because it limits it to an image or words that define what love is. Therefore, if the mind believes love as kind and giving, then that's what we want in someone we fall in love with. What if we believe love is only heartbreak? These misconceptions and limitations don't allow the mind to experience divine love unless it becomes still and untethered. The true love within is mirroring itself outward to the world, while at the same time reflecting the universal love outside of us inward. It is the connection of all love energy through everyone for everyone everywhere.

This is all-encompassing love, which from a higher level doesn't need to be shared with anyone because they also possess it. You can't fill a cup that is already full. In this state there is no more "I" or "you," or any identifiable outer object to be called by individual names. There is no need to understand or grasp anything, because our mind is silent and just observing its experiences. There are no more opinions or words necessary when one experiences this state of being. When the body and mind have witnessed this kind of pure love, then never again do they want to experience anything less.

One day I was consulting and guiding a client who has been meditating for the last forty-five years. We were speaking about what it's like to do the practice and how much had changed in her life. So we went through some of her daily routine, and my intuition said to ask her who she had been practicing with forty-five years ago. It tuned out she had been a disciple of Maharishi Mahesh Yogi, the yogi the Beatles went to India to meet.

I asked: "Did Maharishi give you a mantra?" and she replied yes. "And have you been practicing the same mantra for all these years?" She hadn't. She had been using the mantra sometimes while also using other ones she had been given by random teachers she had met along her path.

For those who are not familiar with *guru diksha*, it means when your guru gives you a mantra. Within this mantra is the energy of pure love. It contains all you need, because your guru knows what you need, as they are connected to the source. So I next asked my client: "Do you remember getting this mantra and how you felt?"

"Pure love." She was given pure love through her mantra, but she got distracted with other mantras, which were also great but not designated for her.

I told her that she needed to resume using her first mantra and following her first guru, as they are both very alive with shakti, the divine power, and need focusing on so she can feel that pure love again. It is a pure love that was offered and given to transform the self, and this comes through as a result of getting the mind out of the way with a practice such as a mantra or meditation.

The Sacrifice for Love

Sacrifice to most people means to give something up. To others it means to give an offering as a ritual. Here sacrifice means to transform: to transform lower superficial love into higher true love; to sacrifice our lower self, to emerge as our higher Self. We sacrifice our lower mind and senses through inner rituals of spiritual practice in order to move past all limitations of this outer life. We still exist in the world, but we don't get involved and become affected by everything around us.

With this approach, sacrifice becomes its true meaning—to be sacred. Sacred love is the source of all consciousness and beyond. It is what breaks past all illusions to what is eternally real. Because we are speaking of energy, this vibration flows without interruptions and at the highest frequency. It is like eating the unseen pure essence of a plant or food and not just taking in the rough and denser part. The essence holds all the power and energy of the plant that is not visible. With love it is the same. The essence of love is not visible but its effects are.

True love or love from the divine is an experience from within that expresses itself outward toward all other living beings. As light attracts light, love attracts love. This is why when we connect in this pure form of love from within we don't have the need or urge to find love with someone outside of ourselves. We realize we are already connected to the source of love and feel fulfilled. At this highest level we are in the most beautiful and fulfilling relationship inwardly. We are joining in soul's love and not mind's ideas of love. So we do not lose ourselves in love but lose our smaller self identity in the bigger Self.

The common outer love most people experience or are searching for takes someone else or something to complete the love circle. When you become aware of the divine love within, you no longer experience love as giving or receiving. Rather, you realize that you keep the connectivity of love between and with everyone by staying within its energy.

You are both love conductor and love supplier. You give it out and allow it to pass through you without holding on to it. It is in trying to hold on to it that we lose love's power. Love is like the river that is flowing and never stops. It flows until there is a diversion or a dam to stop the flow of water. When we are emotional, we create diversions for our love energy. When we are angry, we block the flow altogether. But the water is still moving and trying to find a way through, even though we have put up a blockade. And love is ever present as the water is, no matter what our state of mind. We can deny the presence of love or think that we have stopped loving, but love is still present and alive all around us.

When we are in this conscious dimension and not in the mind, we find ourselves in love with all beings no matter who or what they are. We differentiate between feelings coming from our emotions and mind and the pure love that flows from within. Because pure love doesn't think or feel, it has no discrimination or judgment of people's actions no matter what someone has done. On the mind and sense level, we have preferences that dictate feelings toward one thing or another, toward one person or another. On the highest level, we have no preferences, and we recognize all people as love itself, so hate or conflict can never find a place in our life. We understand that others cannot be any different than we are even if their actions show otherwise.

At this level, all separation is just an illusion we have created from our mind-set and memory. If we do see differences we only see them on the surface level and never at the root of a person's being. How can God have a preference or dislike for God? People's reasoning for peace or war is never coming out of love. They are just concepts of the mind with its own agenda.

As we act more from our perfect spirit or divine nature, we will also have the tendency to start sacrificing outer things. We develop the urge to give away more so nothing disturbs or distracts our state of love. Accumulating becomes burdensome to our mind, which wants to experience love. We start to experience beauty in simplicity, and in turn this brings on more peace and connectivity. We then naturally sacrifice our mind to the divine so it can be tamed and transformed. There is no other way to transcend the mind and move above and beyond it if this transformation doesn't take place. Once you have tasted real, pure love, all other so-called expressions or ideas of love become irrelevant and tasteless.

Shiva/Shakti: Love in a Relationship

If love is the divine—comes from the divine to be shared with the divine—then where does a relationship with another human being fit into this order? We've all heard someone say, "I have to first love myself before understanding how to love someone else." This is a very true statement when coming from the heart and not the mind. When this is stated from the mind, it is from the ego identity. When coming from the heart, this is no longer a statement of want but an admission that we must surrender the mind so love can shine through us.

When two people first notice each other, appearances, looks, and how someone acts are the first things that get our attention. This is like noticing the icing on the cake before tasting it. The next step is exploring and getting to know the other through our senses and mind. This is when we first experience the different flavors, layers, and textures of the other person, just like with the cake.

When the encounters evolve into the beginnings of a relationship, we start to feel more comfortable and show more of our guarded self. Once the relationship has been going for a little while, we are now fully exposed and naked for the other to see "who" we are. But this "who" we are is not our pure Self. From a spiritual standpoint, the relationship is still on the surface level, predominantly under the mind's control. It focuses on the likes and dislikes or psyche of a person at best, which is why it can feel as if we are having the deepest connection with someone, but sometime later we realize we don't know the person at all.

Electricity is a current, and a current is energy. Love is just a current of energy. It doesn't change and become something else because it is running through different homes. We can't have love for someone and not for another. To be in love with all beings requires heart energy and not the intellect. When we are unconditionally in love with all beings—without exception of who they are, where they come from, or what they have done— we will then also be able to maintain a true, loving, and fulfilling relationship with all and everyone, with a spouse or partner, because we will be practicing acceptance with no judgment of what they say or do. This is the proof that we are in pure love with them.

To love without condition is to love purely. This is the kind of love for someone who has done something kind and selfless, and the same love for another who has done something horrible or painful; someone you see as a friend and one you see as an enemy. Have you experienced this pure, untainted love yet? Are you willing to let go of all your "mind stuff" to rise into this love?

You see in this state of being no part of the mind is involved. The mind that thinks, "Well, what about rapists, terrorists, or murderers? Do we still love them after what they have done?" If this even comes into the mind then there is no room for pure love existing in our life. It isn't just loving people we feel good about or think are worthy of love. Can we show it in the face of our deepest prejudices or when we are very angry? That is when love shines through the most.

I want to make it clear that what I am discussing here is the highest standard and aim for the purest kind of love, because we can and should. We are living the effects of ordinary, everyday love, and it isn't working for anyone looking for higher, unconditional love. We need to begin questioning the kinds of relationships and love we create and take part in, questioning whether we are aiming for our highest selves and purest love.

Jaima and I share in this love of Shiva/Shakti, which is the balance of male and female within all of us. It's the reason we came together. This balance is achieved when you are aware of the feminine and masculine energies and which part you are offering in each moment of your relationship. The feminine is the creative energy, movement, and nurturing, and the masculine is the stable grounding energy, the energy that brings creative ideas and makes them happen. Balance is about defining roles based on the energy within the relationship so there is clarity without conflict, and each person can express their higher Self abundantly and without limitation.

It is also much simpler to travel the journey of love with another soul that is following the same spiritual path, because you can act more from the heart. If you and your partner, or even your community, practice the same spiritual rituals, then you will all live in this deep and pure untainted love.

Love for the Divine

Moksha means liberation. In this context it's referring to when the divine, or what we call spirit, soul, or God, has no more use for the physical body and begins to assess its exit strategy. It has other places to be and has completed its work in this particular form. It's when the current lifetime has been lived fully and all karmas have been burned through. This is the ultimate destination for each one of us, without exception. This departure can be a conscious one, so we can have some influence as to where the soul passes on to next. This way we are an active part of transitioning and can be fully conscious of it. In this aware state, our focus is on transformation and love, not on our fear of dying. Just because the body is no longer alive doesn't mean we are not still very much conscious and moving on to other forms of existence.

We have to open the mind to understand truths beyond what we see and hear. The mind needs to expand, at least in theoretical terms, to accept that things like love and spirit continue even when the physical body ceases to exist. If we see love in such an expansive manner and without end, we will be drawn inward toward the source of all love.

There are few guarantees in this life, but dropping the body is one we can count on. This journey to our transition and transformation is so feared because it is misunderstood as an ending. It is not an ending, which has this terrible finale that is forever. It is more about crossroads, other journeys and paths where the soul needs to pick up new tools to be able to continue to help it along to its next destination. It is comparable to the energy of *kundalini* that needs to rise through the *shushumna* (the channel that runs along the spinal column) on its way up to the top of the head. This energy first needs to pass through each of the six chakras to get to the top. At each chakra, or energy point, kundalini is transformed a little more to be able to move on and reach the next chakra. Without the next chakra providing the transformational tools and guidance, the kundalini energy would not be able to reach the top chakra, or *sahasrara,* which is its ultimate destination.

This is the same for our soul or spirit. It is using this body we are in now to transport, transit, and transform itself to the ultimate destination it is transitioning to. Each time the soul takes on a form, it is like a vehicle, a bus or a car. If it reaches a river, then it needs a boat, so it drops the car and continues on this new mode of transportation. So our body, which contains the pure love energy of the soul, is in transit, and at the perfect moment it will not need this body any longer and will trade it in for a new one. Essentially, we are souls in transit with a long layover on earth.

Remember, our soul or spirit is energy, and this energy, being a piece of the whole cosmic consciousness, is located in our heart chakra, or *anahata*. It is our inner yogi that has all the knowledge of the universe—outer and inner. It is beyond death or destruction, beyond all time and space. It is a drop of the divine that eventually makes its way back to the ocean of pure divinity. Our work is to allow this process to happen purposefully and fluidly while being guided during the journey. This is how the mind shows its love for the divine, by assisting and prostrating itself before it so it can pass without resistance.

But this journey is far from peaceful or simple in the world we have manifested. Through living a material existence and forgetting our spiritual path, we have built ourselves a lifestyle in the outside world that has taken our attention away from the inner universe. We are looking outside of our house while we are still inside. Our gaze is pointing outward, being entertained and distracted by our outer environment, while our inner life is calling us. This is indicative of the health and mind issues our society is enduring. We eat and drink what we like, entertain our minds with whatever we desire, speak and act in whatever way we decide. And with all this "freedom" has come much suffering and stress.

We have come to earth to serve our inner master, who is trying to guide our mind to the meaningful and purposeful life we are seeking. The majority of people I encounter are looking for this elusive meaning of life and purposeful living, for love and the higher path. The only ones who are not searching are the very few who have a daily spiritual practice that roots them in the divine. I am not speaking about a few minutes of meditation or yoga asana practice. I'm speaking about practice that roots us so the mind is detached and the inner voice of divinity can be heard. I'm speaking of practice that systematically goes through the different levels of our mind and being to control each one, so when we arrive and fall into meditation there is no more "we" and only "it." A place where there is no more thought or opinion but only release and surrender.

It's a place where we realize that we have not come to earth to play and amuse our senses or minds. We have a deep understanding that our body has a very limited time to do the work we have come here to do. A sense of urgency takes over, in which we feel there is no room for idle talk or conversation that doesn't lead us to our ultimate destination. We realize that each breath we take is like a mantra, which is a part of an even greater expanse of the earth's lungs and the universal tune. With these realizations comes a sense of unity and love for all living entities on earth, but not a mental attachment to them. In this state there is no separation, as there is no mind to analyze or conclude anything beyond what is.

When we reach this state of being, we see death as an exchange in which we go from one life into another, dressed in a new body or outer layer, but that life continues for ages and eras. We see that love continues and spreads beyond our body and into the universe of all consciousness. We are no longer bound by the limited mind but by our limitless divine nature. We no longer fear time or the lack of it. Time becomes irrelevant and unimportant. Our focus shifts from the limited and transient outer world to our inner endless universe, understanding that all the other soul travelers are also on this journey beyond the material form.

There are many celebrations going on in the universe, and we are invited to them all. Transportation is provided to get there, and for each we get to change our attire. All we need to do is enjoy the journey and fulfill our purpose by attending, and then leave once the party is over, so we can get some rest before the next journey begins. This is our spiritual destiny of love from one level to the next. Can you think of a more fun and amazing time than partying around the universe fulfilling our spiritual destiny? I can't.

Chapter Summary

- Love is not a feeling but a state of being.
- Love has no prejudices or preferences.

- Love is not selective or exclusive to a relationship or friendship.
- Love of an enemy demonstrates pure love, as it is much harder to practice.
- Showing love through actions of kindness is more potent than saying "I love you."

Daily Life Practice

1. Every time you think of something you don't like, or have something negative to say about someone, remember you are not practicing love. Become aware and change your perspective until you connect in love with them.

2. Think about strong feelings you have for someone. Now see if you would feel the same if they didn't behave in a way you like. Practice acceptance to the point you feel comfortable, but not to the point you feel resentment. This takes practice.

3. Think of someone you are not fond of, or a group of people you consider yourself separate from or that you have nothing in common with. Now expand your heart and focus on something you do have in common with the person or group.

4. See who and what you are attached to most. Let go a little at a time so they can be free and you can be lighter and have less fear of losing them. This makes for a much deeper love, and most important, fearless relationships.

5. Look to see if your relationship is one of Shiva/Shakti and balanced in like energies. See if you are in a loving and kind relationship that is balanced in responsibilities and duties, one that is feeding you while you feed it. Work to see what you can do to make your relationship more whole.

6. Contemplate universal love and what that might be like. Look at people with deep affection, and don't be disappointed when they do something unacceptable to you or when they let you down. It is in overcoming great disappointments and conflicts that we often arrive at the most beautiful moments of love.

7. If you are single, you can still live in a Shiva/Shakti relationship by balancing your masculine and feminine energy within so that outwardly you are living a balanced and loving life with all beings. Remember that we are in relationships and friendships with all beings and not just exclusively with one.

What Do You Really Want?

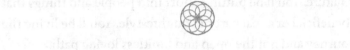

I like to ask my clients, "What do you really want?" Most of the time, they are not very clear and tend to give answers like: "I want to be happy, healthy, sleep well, focus better," a lot of "I want this or that."

I guide them to focus on the bigger picture, which is: "What do you want under all the things you say you want? What do you secretly or silently yearn for?" This gets them thinking of why they get up in the morning or what they dream about at night. It cuts through all the surface thoughts and reveals their deepest desires.

I need to know this key bit of information so I can guide them in the right direction. But they also need to know this deeper yearning about themselves so they won't waste time on things that are distracting, and instead get right to working on the things that really matter. So I am going to ask you the same question: "What do you really want?"

You need to know the answer to this question before moving

forward. If this isn't clear from the start, you will waste many years on things that you really didn't want—things like a relationship that is not based on love, or work that won't allow you to thrive based on your nature. You'll be putting effort into people and things that are not beneficial or a real part of your lifestyle. You'll be living the fearful journey and not the open and limitless loving path.

Once you are clear about this question, then move forward and start to build a routine for yourself that reflects the real lifestyle you envision. If coffee is a part of that lifestyle, then drink coffee. If alcohol is not part of that routine, then put it aside. If playing sports is a part of your lifestyle, then make sure not to just talk about it but to play sports a few times a month. If you are aiming for balance, then balance your time among your family, work, and leisure.

The foundation of your routine will be supported by your daily spiritual practice. This is the backbone of your entire life. It is what gives you support and insight when everything is going well and when it is falling apart. It is what brings clarity in the most confusing and conflicting times. It is the bond and structure that holds together your body and mind when you are struck with illness. It is the light that you can turn on at any time of day or night to guide you.

With this foundation you are then ready to ask the question: "Who am I and why am I?" When you have a fluid routine and lifestyle supported by daily spiritual practice you are ready to ask the bigger questions in life, which won't be answered by the mind but by your higher intuition and heart. You will have the courage to follow your heart even when the guidance is very challenging. With this clarity and deeper understanding that you are the mind on a mental level and spirit on a spiritual level, you will be ready to know your intentions and what motivates you to take the actions you take and behave the way you do.

With this insight you will be able to see every intention you have with clarity, and shift and change the ones that are no longer part of your lifestyle. The lifestyle you have decided to live dictates what your intentions are and what you want to attract into your life.

From all this work you have put in to control the mind and create balanced habits, you will come closer to understanding and seeing what your true purpose is, what your mind has made up as a purpose and what your spirit's life purpose is. The distinction between the two will be clear at this stage, because your mind will have desire- and sense-oriented purposes, while the soul will have a much higher, challenging purpose. Both are valid, but the higher path will now be something you want to spend more time exploring, if not starting to live and move toward with precise actions and decisions.

At this stage of our development service to all beings becomes a natural feeling, attitude, and way of life. Giving and the mentality of being one with others is not something we need to look for anymore but becomes what we are.

The culmination of all this work naturally brings us to feel divine love. What we are feeling is not separate from us and doesn't come from anyplace but the heart. These yogic practices are the steps, the journey, and the path that lead us to the heart, where we find the source of all of creation.

We cannot get there without doing this work daily, because the world outside is constantly pulling at us and distracting our mind to fall out of balance. Ancient sages knew we would need help in these times and therefore set out this foolproof way of spiritual living, so our mind could be used in the fullest and best possible way.

Everyone has the potential to reach their goals, but the goal needs to be defined and then reached through effort and discipline, becoming a joyful journey of learning, but one that also has difficult and tough times. It is through these challenging times that we experience our most valuable lessons, which serve us throughout our life.

Remember, we don't learn much from easy times. We show our character and determination through the most arduous times, bringing us the greatest rewards. Aim high! It's a better investment. Anytime my mind starts to complain that this work is hard, I reflect on a life that doesn't have these grounding practices and a routine built on the higher Self, and immediately I am pulled back into the heart, feeling gratitude, bliss, and love for all there is in this life. Becoming aware and conscious of higher living is a blessing.

To kick-start your Yogi Code Routine and Practice, I've laid out a twenty-one-day plan, which integrates many of the practices in this book plus some new ones. The intention behind this plan is to establish a good foundational routine while you meditate and work on your intentions, creating a lifestyle that supports your path in life.

I know this takes time and contemplation to perfect, and this twenty-one-day yogi code kick-start will guide you through and give you the support you need to be able to continue for many years to come. You can either adapt all the practices into your life routine or take practices one at a time, adding in more as you go along. But make sure that the five Yogi Code Practices in chapter 3 are always a part of your life, every morning—the foundation from which to build upon.

I have seen amazing things happen for people living the seven Yogi Code laws taught in this book and discovering their inner yogi. I want you to also experience these amazing life changes. I hope you do too!

Appendix: Twenty-One-Day
Yogi Code Kick-Start

This is a twenty-one-day kick-start plan to motivate you to do your Yogi Code Practices and then continue to practice beyond as a lifelong pursuit. More videos and tutorials can be found at YCMembership.com.

The first five practices are from the section titled "Your Yogi Code Practice" in chapter 3. These are your foundational practices, to be performed each morning to ground your mind and body in order for you to focus and set great intentions for the day. This is your spiritual practice that you do regardless of whether you choose to do any other practice.

Once you have integrated this morning practice each day, then add a Daily Life Practice to your routine from the twenty-one-day plan, which will be different each day. Each of these Daily Life Practices in the twenty-one-day plan are meant to be applied throughout your day at breakfast, at work, with family, with friends, or in any situation to give you the opportunity to practice in real-life situations. All of these practices are tools to remind, guide, and assist you to work your way through challenging experiences rather than avoid them.

Let's get started!

Your Yogi Code Practice

Dedicate a space for your practice, burn some incense, and play the tamboura sound (you will find this on YCMembership.com) in the background. Have a mat, rug, hard cushion, or chair to sit on.

These five practices should be the first thing you do after brushing your teeth and bathing. The morning practice will soon become a good habit, creating more great and healthy habits.

Keep your eyes closed during these practices unless otherwise instructed. This will help you go further inward.

1. Full Yogic Breath

- Sit on the floor in a cross-legged position (if your knees are off the floor, sit on a hard, solid cushion or blankets until your knees are further down than your hips) or sit in a chair with your spine straight.

- Start to inhale, first feeling the stomach expand outward. Then the rib cage expands and then the chest, in this order. When exhaling, first feel the chest deflate, then the rib cage, and finally the stomach. To exhale fully, pull the stomach in all the way without straining until all the air has been exhaled from the lungs.
- Inhale again, expanding stomach, rib cage, and chest. Exhale, deflating the chest, rib cage, and stomach, which is pulled in all the way.
- Make the breath very controlled, slow, and deep so at no time do you force the air in or out quickly and lose control over it.
- Do this practice for three to seven minutes.
- Sit quietly for a moment and see how the practice affects your mind.

2. Humming Bee (*Bhramari*)

- To start the practice, sit in a comfortable seated posture so you are very stable and your back is straight.
- Now bring your arms up, open the elbows outward, and put your index finger into your ears. Don't press your fingers in too hard but also not too lightly.

- Keep the mouth and lips closed, with the teeth a little apart. Inhale very slowly through the nostrils. Exhale through the nose while making a long, even, and steady humming noise. Don't force the breath but do it smoothly. Rest your arms between each round if they become tired; otherwise, do the rounds consecutively.
- Do five rounds.
- Sit quietly for a moment and see how the practice affects your mind.

3. Chakra Purification Focus (*Unmani mudra*)

- Sit in a comfortable seated posture with a straight spine.
- Bring your attention to the back of your head at the top of the spine. Inhale and hold the breath for a second. As you start to exhale, do so in a controlled manner, letting the air out very slowly. As you exhale, visualize your energy descending through the spine (you will be passing through all the chakras) until you reach the bottom of the spine. As you are exhaling and lowering your attention down the spine, your eyes can also be lowering and closing. (If the practice of opening and closing the

eyes doesn't feel right at first, leave it out until you
have more experience with the practice.)
- Hold the breath for a second, then start to inhale
  slowly. As you inhale, bring your attention upward
  through the spine (again, you will be passing
  through all the chakras). As you move upward, your
  eyes also can be opening slowly.
- Repeat this cycle seven times. One cycle is one trip
  down and up through the spine.
- Make sure to move slowly while expanding your
  breath in and out in a controlled manner like you
  did with the full yogic breath.
- After each round you can take a few yogic breaths
  and return to do the next round, or you can do the
  five rounds continuously.
- At the end of all five rounds sit quietly and observe
  the mind.

4. Mantra Aum-OM (*Japa*)

This practice can be done either audibly or silently.

- Sit comfortably and in a grounded position with
  your spine straight.
- Inhale and exhale a few rounds of yogic breath. On
  the next exhale, with open mouth start to chant

Oooooooooo, and three-quarters of the way through the breath, close the lips and continue making the sound *mmmmmmmmmm*.

- Then inhale again and repeat the process for five to seven rounds.
- If you are doing the practice silently, you can recite the mantra OM when inhaling and exhaling if you feel comfortable. Otherwise just chant while exhaling.
- If doing the practice out loud, only repeat the mantra while exhaling.
- When you are finished, sit quietly and observe the mind.

5. Heart Chakra Meditation (*Anahata Dharana*)

- Sit in a comfortable, stable posture where you don't have to move for a while.
- Close your eyes. Bring your index finger and thumb together and turn your palms upward, placing them on your knees. This mudra invokes consciousness when the palms face upward; when facing downward they invoke knowledge.
- Take a full yogic breath. Bring your awareness to the heart area. Keep breathing.

+ Start to silently repeat the mantra YAM. Chant it
  as *Yaaaaaaa-mmmmm*, making the *A* and *M* longer.
  (The *A* is pronounced softly, as though you were
  saying *YUM*.) Keep breathing and slowly repeat.
+ All your focus should be in the heart area in the
  center of the chest. This is also the location of the
  anahata chakra.
+ Keep breathing slowly, repeating YAM and focusing.
+ Do this for five to seven minutes. Don't worry
  about timing it. You will feel when to stop
  intuitively.
+ After the practice, just sit for a moment.
+ Start to listen to the heart.
+ Start to feel the heart.
+ Notice what your message is from the heart, so you
  act on it today.
+ Allow your intuition to guide you. Be open to it by
  surrendering your mind to it.
+ When finishing, bring your awareness or focus from
  the heart and draw the energy all the way up to look
  between your eyebrows at the third eye, or ajna
  chakra, and take a long yogic breath. Close the eyes
  and observe how you are feeling and how the mind
  is. After a few breaths, bring your hands into prayer
  position in front of the heart. You are bowing your

head to the teacher inside and being grateful for all
the guidance it is giving you.

* Remember: if not at this time, many messages and
guidance will be coming to you during the day
through your intuition if you stay tuned in to this
frequency you have created.

The Twenty-One-Day Plan

DAY ONE: PUTTING YOUR BEST FOOT FORWARD

Before you get out of bed, feel and sense from which nostril the air
is flowing more freely.

Step out of bed with the foot that corresponds to the same side
as which nostril is flowing more freely. Stand on that foot and leg
fully while balancing yourself on the ball of the opposite foot.

You are now standing straight on one leg and using the other
foot's toes for balancing the body. Slowly take seven breaths in
and out.

This practice not only helps you be conscious of the very first
step you take out of bed to start your day but is a yogic practice to
align the energy of the mind and body with the earth and universal
vibrations.

DAY TWO: VOCAL ATTENTION

After flossing and brushing your teeth, scrape your tongue with a tongue scraper. Then gargle with some premade sesame oil mixed with a few drops of tea tree oil through the teeth and around the mouth. Do this for a minute or two.

This practice will strengthen the gums and teeth and move excess mucus out of the throat. It's a great practice for making the voice sharp as you look to your day of speaking and communicating.

DAY THREE: CLEANSING THE GATEWAY
TO THE MIND FOR GREATER FOCUS

There are different ways to do this practice. The simplest is to use a neti pot to clean out the nasal cavity of all the excess mucus that has collected from the night's sleep.

Fill your neti pot up with warm water and add a few pinches of salt.

Wash out each nostril once or twice depending on the level of blockage. If you don't have a neti pot, cup your hand and add a little warm water and a tiny bit of salt. Sniff this into one nostril and spit the water out of your mouth. Repeat this on the other side.

DAY FOUR: REFLECTION AND CLOSURE

Sit for a few minutes about sixty to ninety minutes before bed. Don't wait until you are sleepy. You need an alert mind for this practice.

Sit and reflect on your day. What was an action or word you could have changed to make a conversation move smoother? Did you attract what you wanted, or are you attracting people and work you are not energized about? What could you have done better? What needs to change in your attitude or actions to make things go peacefully? This practice is about what changes you can bring to your own actions and not anyone else's. Once you have identified one thing, make sure to take it into your day tomorrow and apply it.

Let your thoughts just be present and know tomorrow is the day when you take better actions, but now it is time for sleep. Prepare yourself for bed.

DAY FIVE

To reach and live a higher state of consciousness, speak less today. See if you can speak with an awakened consciousness. When you do speak, use your words wisely and carefully, so they are kind but direct. Create clarity so people understand you quickly and you don't have to repeat yourself.

DAY SIX

When you wake up in the morning, recall or write in a journal what you dreamed about (as much detail as you can remember). As part of knowing yourself better, you also need to know what the mind is thinking during sleep. Many of our fears and conflicts arise at night. Try to write these down weekly to see if there are patterns of thought that need working through.

DAY SEVEN

Sit for just seven minutes and reflect on the thoughts you are having. What do you know about yourself that you would like to change? Make it clear why you want to change and how you feel this should happen.

DAY EIGHT

Ask yourself: "Who am I?" Then be quiet for a moment and reflect. Doing this over time will take you deeper into contemplation of your higher Self, but you have to ask with love and compassion, as this is the language the heart responds to. It takes practice and patience to get an answer to this question. But you will receive one.

DAY NINE

Make it clear how much are you willing to do to bring your deepest intentions into being. How hard are you willing to work to make your deepest intentions manifest? Are you actively motivated, or are you doubtful or lazy about it? Be honest so you can set realistic goals for yourself without feeling disappointed again and again. Once you know what you are willing to do, take the actions necessary before the mind talks you out of it.

DAY TEN

What do you repeat every day that has become your mantra? "I can," "I will," "when possible," "not now," "sure, soon," or "when I get the time"? Change your mantra today to what it needs to be for you to reach your goal and feel accomplishment and love for all.

DAY ELEVEN

What is the overall intention of your life? Is it to find happiness, to experience joy, to be successful, to be loved, or to be liberated? Today is the day to follow your actions and know the intentions behind them. It's a time to focus on the most important things and let go of nonessential, time-consuming activities.

DAY TWELVE

Do the words you speak match the intentions you have? Today observe how you speak to people and what you tend to say or repeat. Are you genuine, or do you find it difficult to express your thoughts? Is your intention to serve or to get something? Be honest, and be who you are unless you feel you need to change. Being true to ourselves means living out the intentions we have. Make sure your intentions bring you peace and love down the road.

DAY THIRTEEN

Today no matter what or who bothers you, repeat this: "It's just all mind stuff." If someone is arguing with you or is agitated, if they are repeating things or getting confused, just repeat: "It's just mind stuff and it will pass." But only tell yourself, not the other person!

DAY FOURTEEN

Make a point not to waste your sexual creative energy on meaningless sex, talk, or actions, which drain your body and mind. Put all this power into healing, creating, and making things count on a higher level. Pick something of utmost importance and put this creative energy into it.

DAY FIFTEEN

Look into your life and see how you spend most of your time each day. Is there a part of your day when you are being of service? A part of the day you can be more present? Are you giving more importance to your cell phone, social media, or work when you should be listening to a loved one or someone in need? Make a point of doing this today and every day.

DAY SIXTEEN

Today think about how you can make everything you do and say become a service to everyone. See if you can bring the attitude of service into your workplace or home. If this is hard, start with one thing and then silently observe what benefit it has for everyone. Then build on the energy.

DAY SEVENTEEN

Being of service to humanity requires you to expand your mind and let go of the prejudices you have collected from the past. This could be a dislike toward a person or group for what they stand for or for what they are. It could be toward other countries. In being of service, we don't need to go to war to serve but to control the wars in our mind that we burden other people with.

DAY EIGHTEEN

Every time you think of something you don't like or have something negative to say about someone, remember you are not practicing love. Become aware and change your perspective until you connect in love with them. What don't you like about them? Aren't they just like you? If you don't recognize them as yourself, then keep practicing until you and they melt into one.

DAY NINETEEN

Are you in a Shiva/Shakti relationship, a relationship that is balanced in like energies that are traveling on the same path? One that is fulfilling and full of love energy? Make shifts to your relationship by using the material in this book so you can grow more in love together.

If you are single, use the practices in chapter 3 to balance your masculine and feminine energy so you can have a loving relationship with all beings.

DAY TWENTY

See who and what you are attached to most. Let go a little so they can be free and you can be lighter and have less fear of losing them. This makes for a much deeper love, and most important, for a fearless relationship.

DAY TWENTY-ONE

Contemplate universal love and what that might be like. Look at people with deep affection, and don't be disappointed when they do something unacceptable to you or when they let you down. We are not perfect, but love is; let it lead you into having love for all.

Acknowledgments

Amy Hughes, my agent, thank you so much for always being there to support and add your guidance to the path of each book. This time has been no exception. You are wonderful. Zhena Muzyka, my publisher, you are a new light on this journey and such a wonderful one. Thank you for adding all the essential ingredients for making this book become better.

Emily Han, thank you for doing such a masterful job editing the book. You have been such a joy to work with.

Kulin and Dipika Shah from 3rdeye digital marketing, you two do such a professional job of running all the online and social media marketing of the Yogi Cameron brand. I can't thank you enough for all the work you do.

My spiritual brothers, Suresh and Shreesha, you are both great teachers and guides along the yogic path.

Dr. Hari and Ganga, being in satsang with you both is one of my favorite times in life. You are great teachers to all.

My wife, Yogini Jaima, you are my spiritual soul mate and your support and love has been paramount to life having all the beautiful colors and moments it has. Thank you for being you.

Azusena, my amazing daughter, I love the way we laugh together. You are an inspiration to watch as you bring your gift of music to the world.

Theresa, my mother, you are a beautiful soul who has shown my sister, Soraya, and me such love and support throughout our lives. We love you dearly.

Sanskrit Glossary

anahata: The heart chakra, or energy center, located in the heart area.

anandamaya kosha: The sheath of bliss and highest consciousness.

antar kumbhaka: The retention of the breath after inhaling.

ayurveda: The oldest medicinal system in use today.

Bhagavad Gita: A seven-hundred-verse Hindu scripture teaching spiritual wisdom.

bhastrika: The rigorous pushing out and pulling in of the stomach during pranayama practice.

bundha: A lock or holding of energy that is applied to different parts of the body.

chakra: Wheels or energy centers.

dirga swasam: Full breath or three-part breathing.

dharana: Concentration.

dharma: Purpose or life duties.

dualism: To be divided in opposite directions.

guru: A master or one who is enlightened.

jalandhara bandha: A throat lock.

kapalabhati: Rapid diaphragmatic breathing.

karma: Action; when we take an action there is a reaction.

kosha: A sheath or layer.

kriya: Cleansing practices through different techniques.

kumbhaka: The holding or retention of breath.

kundalini: The sexual energy that rises through the chakras toward the top of the head.

mantra: Sacred words and syllables in Sanskrit used for chanting.

moksha: Liberation from the body.

moola bundha: Locking or squeezing the perineum or anus muscle.

mudra: Hand, finger, or body gestures and symbols.

nadi: A channel of the body and mind.

nadi shodhana: Alternate-nostril breathing.

prana: The vital or subtlest part of energy in our body and mind.

pranayama: Control of prana during different practices.

rishi: Sage who is a seer of the past, present, and future. Through meditation they can see everything in the universe.

sadhana: Spiritual practice.

sage: One whom God speaks through to teach all others.

sahasrara: The chakra or energy point at the top of the head.

samana: The air that controls digestion.

sankalpa: Intentions.

satvic: Balanced and pure.

shakti: The female aspect of the divine.

shaktipat: Opening of the third eye through the grace of the guru.

shatkarma: Purification practices done before yoga practice.

Shiva: The male aspect of the divine.

sushumna: The channel that runs along the spinal column.

udana: The air that moves upward in the body.

ujjai: A pranayama practice of constricting the throat while breathing very slowly.

upana: The downward movement of air in the body.

vata: The element of air.

vayana: The air that moves to the extremities of the body.

Vedas: Ancient Hindu scriptures of knowledge and practice.

yantra: Meditative ritual geometric shape.

yogi: One who practices the yogic path.

yuga: An age or era.

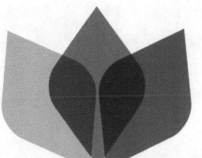

ENLIVEN ™

About Our Books: We are the world's first holistic publisher for mission-driven authors. We curate, create, collaborate on, and commission sophisticated, fresh titles and voices to enhance your spiritual development, success, and wellness pursuits.

About Our Vision: Our authors are the voice of empowerment, creativity, and spirituality in the twenty-first century. You, our readers, are brilliant seekers of adventure, unexpected stories, and tools to transform yourselves and your world. Together, we are change-makers on a mission to increase literacy, uplift humanity, ignite genius, and create reasons to gather around books. We think of ourselves as instigators of soulful exchange.

Welcome to the wondrous world of Enliven Books, a new imprint from Zhena Muzyka, author of *Life by the Cup: Inspiration for a Purpose-Filled Life*, and Atria, an imprint of Simon & Schuster, Inc.

To explore our list of books and learn about fresh new voices in the realm of Mind-Body-Spirit, please visit us at

EnlivenBooks.com | **/EnlivenBooks**